Sexuality, Politic
AIDS in Brazı

Social Aspects of AIDS

Series Editor: Peter Aggleton
Goldsmiths' College, University of London

Sexuality, Politics and AIDS in Brazil
In Another World?

Herbert Daniel and Richard Parker

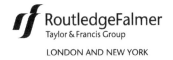

RoutledgeFalmer
Taylor & Francis Group

LONDON AND NEW YORK

First published in 1993
by RoutledgeFalmer
2 Park Square, Milton Park, Abingdon, Oxon, OX14 4RN

Transferred to Digital Printing 2006

**A catalogue record for this book is available from the British
Library**

ISBN 0 75070 135 8
ISBN 0 75070 136 6 pbk

Jacket design by Caroline Archer
Typeset in 11/13pt Bembo by
Graphicraft Typesetters Ltd, Hong Kong

Publisher's Note
The publisher has gone to great lengths to ensure the quality of this
reprint but points out that some imperfections in the original may be
apparent

This book is the product of 'quatro mãos' (four hands). It was in the final stages of completion when Herbert Daniel died on 29 March 1992. It is dedicated to Claudio Mesquita, Daniel's partner in life for more than twenty years.

Contents

Contents

Series Editor's Preface

It is increasingly recognized that research into sexual meanings, sexual identities and sexual cultures is essential if HIV and AIDS health promotion activities are to be well founded. For to ignore the various ways in which people interpret and understand their sexual lives is to run the risk of devising culturally inappropriate and ineffective interventions. Likewise, the insights and experience of those living with HIV disease are essential if we are to be effective in challenging deep seated prejudices and hostilities. This insight is vital too for the development of a more constructive politics of AIDS — a politics which challenges efforts to marginalize, stigmatize and discriminate, and one which insists on the involvement of people with HIV disease in activities related to prevention and care.

All of these concerns are central to the arguments in this book. Drawing upon nearly a decade's experience, Herbert Daniel and Richard Parker chart the course of the epidemic and its social effects in Brazil. The analysis they offer is rigorous, incisive and compelling, and derives both from social scientific research and personal involvement in community activism around AIDS. The authors portray graphically what it means to live with AIDS in contemporary Brazil, and how the epidemic has impacted upon the lives of individuals and communities.

Pointing to the inadequacy of Western models as a way of understanding the effects of the epidemic, *Sexuality, Politics and AIDS in Brazil* argues for a more sophisticated appreciation of the ways in which sexuality is understood and lived. While its focus is on sexual behaviour between men, and male sexual desire, the analysis developed has more general applicability. It highlights, for example, the limits of attempts to understand the social dynamics of HIV and AIDS in 'outsider' terms — be these the categories offered by mainstream epidemiology or those imposed by government or state bureaucracies. *Sexuality, Politics and*

AIDS in Brazil points too to global inequalities in health and their impact on individuals and communities. It makes available to a wider readership ideas central to the development of a more critical and reflexive HIV and AIDS health promotion practice.

Peter Aggleton

Note on Translation and Language

Throughout this text many Portuguese terms and expressions have been maintained in referring to key cultural categories such as the classifications of Brazilian sexual culture. In addition, English-language terms have sometimes been adopted which might strike many readers as at least somewhat unexpected. This is particularly true, for example, in the use of the term 'homosexual' (following common usage in Brazilian Portuguese, and as opposed to the more common use of 'gay' in English) throughout much of the text. It should go without saying that the goal of such usage is in no way to suggest a preference for one or another type of terminology, but, on the contrary, consistently to draw the reader's attention to issues of cross-cultural difference.

Acknowledgments

We wish to thank the following for permission to republish revised versions of these essays:

Greenwood Press for 'Responding to AIDS in Brazil' (Chapter 1 in this volume), first published in Barbara A. Misztal and David Moss (eds), *Action on AIDS: National Policies in Comparative Perspective*, New York, Greenwood Press, 1990.

Editora Iglu for 'AIDS no Brazil: A Falência dos Modelos' (Chapter 2 in this volume), first published in Herbert Daniel and Richard Parker, *AIDS: A Terceira Epidemia*, São Paulo, Editora Iglu, 1991.

The Panos Institute for 'The Third Epidemic: An Exercise in Solidarity' (Chapter 3 in this volume), first published in *The Third Epidemic: Repercussions of the Fear of AIDS*, London, Panos Institute, 1990.

The American Anthropological Association for 'Acquired Immunodeficiency Syndrome in Urban Brazil' (Chapter 4 in this volume), *Medical Anthropology Quarterly*, new series, 1, 155–175.

The International Union for the Scientific Study of Population for 'Male Prostitution, Bisexual Behaviour and HIV Transmission in Urban Brazil' (Chapter 5 in this volume), first published in Tim Dyson (ed.), *Sexual Behaviour and Networking: Anthropological and Socio-Cultural Studies on the Transmission of HIV*, Liège, Editions Derouaux-Ordina, 1992.

Editora Iglu for 'Depois da AIDS: Mudanças no Comportamento (Homos)sexual' (Chapter 6 in this volume), first published in Herbert Daniel and Richard Parker, *AIDS: A Terceira Epidemia*, São Paulo, Editora Iglu, 1991.

Oxford University Press for 'AIDS Education and Health Promotion in Brazil: Lessons from the Past and Prospects for the Future' (Chapter 7 in this volume), first published in Jaime Sepulveda, Harvey Fineberg and Jonathan Mann (eds), *AIDS Prevention through Education: A World View*, New York, Oxford University Press, 1992.

The Brazilian Interdisciplinary AIDS Association for 'Notícias da Outra Vida' (Chapter 8 in this volume), first published in Herbert Daniel, *A Vida Antes da Morte*, Rio de Janeiro, Jaboti, 1989.

The Brazilian Interdisciplinary AIDS Association for 'Antes, A Vida' (Chapter 9 in this volume), first published in Herbert Daniel, *A Vida Antes da Morte*, Rio de Janeiro, Jaboti, 1989.

The Brazilian Interdisciplinary AIDS Association for 'AIDS: O Imobilismo do Medo e a Resposta da Solidariedade' (Chapter 10 in this volume), presented at the Rights and Humanity Workshop, Haia, 1991.

Editora Iglu for 'O Primeiro AZT a Gente Nunca Esquece' (Chapter 11 in this volume), published in Herbert Daniel and Richard Parker, *AIDS: A Terceira Epidemia*, São Paulo, Editora Iglu, 1991.

The Brazilian Interdisciplinary AIDS Association for 'A Alma do Cidadão' (Chapter 12 in this volume), presented at the Eighth International Conference on AIDS, 1991.

In addition, we would particularly like to thank the Wenner-Gren Foundation for Anthropological Research, the Joint Committee on Latin American Studies of the Social Science Research Council and the American Council of Learned Societies, with funds provided by the National Endowment for the Humanities and the Ford Foundation, the Social and Behavioural Research Unit of the World Health Organization's Global Programme on AIDS, and the Foundation for the Support of Research in the State of Rio de Janeiro (FAPERJ) for their support of Richard Parker's research on the social dimensions of AIDS in Brazil, and the Ford Foundation and the Inter-American Foundation for their support of Herbert Daniel's work as a writer with the Brazilian Interdisciplinary AIDS Association (ABIA). Without the generous support of these diverse institutions it is unlikely that the texts that comprise this book could have been produced.

Finally, our special thanks to Vagner de Almeida and Claudio Mesquita for their constant support, to João Guerra, Cesar Behs, Jane Galvão, José Stalin Pedrosa and Herbert de Souza for their diverse contributions to this work, and to Susana Alvino, Lys France Portella, and Lilia Rossi for their assistance in the preparation of the manuscript and their help in resolving all manner of problems in day-to-day life.

Introduction

Herbert Daniel and Richard Parker

Perhaps more than anything else, this volume represents an attempt to cross boundaries. It emerges from our own desire to overcome at least some of the divisions that, in our opinion, have limited the ways in which the world community has thought about and analyzed HIV and AIDS — the ways in which it has sought to respond to the international AIDS pandemic.

Much like our first book together, *AIDS: A Terceira Epidemia* [*AIDS: The Third Epidemic*], which was published in Portuguese in 1991, this collection of essays was born from what we describe as an interdisciplinary affair. In it the perspectives of an American anthropologist and a Brazilian writer meet one another in seeking to understand the social reactions that have emerged in response to the AIDS epidemic — reactions created more often than not by what we would describe as an ideological virus whose consequences have often been more dangerous and even deadly than the epidemic caused by the biological virus known as HIV.

When we first met, brought together by the epidemic itself, initially in 1985 and then again in 1988, what we describe as the night-time drama of HIV/AIDS seemed very dark indeed. It was a night characterized above all else by the widespread prejudice and discrimination which seemed to be the only backdrop for the epidemic and its sick. It was here, within this scenery, that the degradation of those considered to be the preferential targets of the epidemic was assured — at first, particularly, behaviourally homosexual and bisexual men, and, as time passed, other similarly 'marginal' groups. Quarantine. Isolation. Stigmatization. Violence. Murder. The shadows of a night at once ominous and oppressive.

Through long hours of conversation we began to build not only a profound friendship but a common understanding of the epidemic

1

and the threats it posed. Working together on a range of projects, we began to find small glimpses of clarity within the darkness. At the same time we learned that such clarity would be almost invisible to the cold eye of science seeking to be exact — that it is born, on the contrary, from the very movements of gestation within society itself.

The reactions to HIV/AIDS provoked by panic and alarm were, in general, stimulated by grossly distorted visions of the epidemic — visions which resulted in the immobilization of many governments and social institutions. Yet against this and in spite of this, there also emerged another very different response, in general consolidated in community organizations. Born of the most varied initiatives and within diverse communities around the globe, such organizations have developed innovative and mobilizing conceptions about the epidemic and have developed more adequate responses to the challenges it poses. It is principally about these conceptions and responses that we have written in the essays that make up this volume.

At the same time, in focusing on such issues within the specific context of the society where we live and work, in Brazil, we have also sought to raise for English-language readers the question of cultural difference as crucial to any attempt to understand or address the HIV/AIDS epidemic internationally. Just as the forces of hope and solidarity, like those of prejudice and discrimination, exhibit a certain universality (making it possible, however tentatively, to bridge the boundaries of society and culture), they simultaneously take shape and exist within social and cultural situations that are characterized more by difference and diversity than by sameness or similarity.

In the essays that make up this volume we try to call attention to such differences, to the particularities and specificities that characterize, in this case, Brazilian life. With this in mind, we have divided the book into three major sections. In the first, as a way of introducing the reader both to Brazil and to the peculiarities of the HIV/AIDS epidemic that has taken shape there, we have included essays focusing in different ways on the social construction of AIDS in Brazil. In the second we turn more specifically to the question of sexuality, and to the particularities of the sexual culture that we believe to be crucial not only to an understanding of the epidemiology of HIV transmission in Brazil, but also as a foundation for the development of AIDS prevention programs. Finally, in the third section we look at the ways in which Brazilian society has responded to the epidemic — at what it means to live with HIV/AIDS in Brazil in the late twentieth century.

The texts comprising these different sections are themselves diverse, marked by the very different backgrounds and styles of their authors.

The relative caution and constant qualification of a North American social scientist contrast sharply, for example, with the much more poetic, absolute and even, at times, didactic style of a Brazilian novelist and political activist writing from within a very different discursive tradition. Yet, for all their differences, the texts meet and even intertwine, we believe, through their constant focus on the particularities and details of Brazilian life, and on the implications of such details for our understanding of HIV and AIDS.

By focusing on the particularities that characterize each of the major areas that we examine in this book — particularities that profoundly determine the very shape and structure of the HIV/AIDS epidemic in Brazil, as well as the ways in which Brazilian society has sought to respond to it — we hope to build the way, increasingly, for the comparative analysis of cross-cultural difference that we believe must ultimately provide the foundation not only for a more effective global response to the international AIDS pandemic, but for a fuller understanding of our shared experience as human beings. It is only by placing the particularities of social and cultural life within a comparative perspective, by establishing an analytic tension between similarity and difference across social and cultural boundaries, that the forces which at once divide and unite us globally begin to become intelligible. It is only through the understanding that such mutual reflection makes possible that our common predicament becomes meaningful.

Ultimately, it is the capacity to recognize difference, and to respect it, that lies at the heart of human solidarity. It is such solidarity, based upon a respect for difference, we believe, that offers not only the most effective vaccine against HIV/AIDS, but the blueprint for structuring the edifice of a better world.

Part 1

The Social Construction of AIDS in Brazil

Chapter 1

AIDS in Brazil

Richard Parker

Since the earliest confirmed cases began to be registered in 1982 and 1983, the rapid spread of HIV infection and AIDS in Brazil has become increasingly evident (see, for example, *Folha de São Paulo*, 1986; Panos Institute, 1988; Rodrigues and Chequer, 1987). By 1986 the number of reported cases of AIDS in Brazil had surpassed the numbers reported by countries such as France and Haiti, and since that time, even with increased reporting from the nations of central Africa, Brazil has consistently ranked among the leaders on the list of nations reporting cases to the World Health Organization (see, for example, Rodrigues and Chequer, 1987; see also Chapter 4 in this volume). Indeed, by mid-1992, after more than a decade of unchecked expansion, for reasons that will become clearer later, the epidemic had spread to every region of the country, and as many as 28,455 cases and 12,873 confirmed deaths had been reported to the Brazilian Ministry of Health (see Table 1). Even more troubling, while reliable seroprevalence data have been extremely limited and the analysis of epidemiological tendencies has thus had to rely largely upon case reporting, the Ministry of Health estimated that as many as 700,000 to 1,000,000 Brazilians may already be infected with HIV as the AIDS epidemic enters its second decade in Brazil.

In spite of such statistics, however, the AIDS epidemic in Brazil has been the focus of relatively limited attention. Discussion of the international AIDS pandemic has tended to focus, on the contrary, on a small number of better known cases or examples that have then been taken as almost paradigmatic in constructing an understanding of the global dimensions of HIV infection and AIDS (see Treichler, 1992). Not only media representations, but even epidemiological models and scientific discourse have tended to emphasize what are perceived as the extremes of social and cultural difference, focusing (almost always superficially), in particular, on AIDS in the United States or in the countries of central Africa, and building upon these cases a particular vision of the international dimensions of the epidemic (see Patton, 1991; Treichler, 1992). More ambiguous, or less clearly contrastable, examples have largely escaped significant attention, and have generally been dismissed as curious exceptions or perplexing footnotes within the more orthodox description of the epidemic.

Yet it is perhaps precisely because of this tendency that a closer examination of the Brazilian case (like others that in one way or another seem to fall outside the boundaries of both the familiar and the exotic) is especially instructive. Precisely because the AIDS epidemic in Brazil fails to fit neatly into existing paradigms — because it seems to combine a range of contrasting features, and thus to take shape as a kind of hybrid, not only of epidemiological patterns but of social and cultural forces and reactions — it forces us to re-examine many of the central assumptions that have dominated the discussion of AIDS internationally. To begin to develop an understanding of the HIV/AIDS epidemic in Brazil, we are forced to move beyond such assumptions, to deconstruct the images that have been built up around the epidemic, both within Brazilian culture itself as well as in the international imagery of AIDS, and to focus on the particularities and details of Brazilian life. Ultimately, it is this exercise in what I would describe as 'close reading' (see Geertz, 1973) — this focus on the local and the particular, on the specific social, cultural, political and economic factors that have shaped not only the epidemiology of AIDS in Brazil, but also the social and cultural reactions and responses to the epidemic — that might then permit us to move back, beyond preconceived notions and unexamined assumptions, to a fuller understanding of the AIDS pandemic more generally, and of the ways in which this pandemic has taken shape cross-culturally.

The Changing Shape of the Epidemic

Although cases of AIDS had begun to be diagnosed in Brazil as early as 1982, relatively little public attention was given to a disease that was perceived as afflicting only the wealthy homosexual population of the United States (see Trevisan, 1986). It was not until June 1983, with the death of a leading fashion designer, that AIDS began to draw the attention of the Brazilian media (see Chapter 4 in this volume; Perlongher, 1987b; Panos Institute, 1988; Trevisan, 1986). Even then, however, because the designer, like the other early cases, was himself a well known and well-to-do homosexual who spent much of his time in

New York, the focus of this increasing attention was directed less at understanding the disease than at classifying and categorizing its so-called victims.

Even before AIDS had become statistically significant in Brazil, then, it had become the subject of media attention and, by extension, a topic of conversation in daily life (see Chapters 2 and 3 in this volume; Morães and Carrara, 1985). Playing on a complex, and sometimes contradictory, set of beliefs related to emotionally charged subjects such as sexuality and death, the discussion of the disease was almost invariably carried out less in terms of objective knowledge of scientific information than in terms of misinformation or partial information (ABIA, 1988a). Between 1983 and 1985 an image of AIDS and its perceived victims was gradually constructed in Brazilian popular culture that was only loosely based on available epidemiological information, but that would prove to be perhaps the most powerful force shaping the Brazilian response to the epidemic for years to come. Throughout this period the vast majority of people with HIV/AIDS were thought to be well-to-do individuals who enjoyed the luxury of dividing their time between Rio de Janeiro or São Paulo and foreign centres such as New York or Paris. Even more important, they were almost uniformly identified as homosexual males whose sexual conduct was characterized by its high degree of promiscuity. The extent to which this image of the so-called AIDS victim as a wealthy, promiscuous, homosexual male in fact represented epidemiological reality was rarely raised, even by medical experts and public health officials, as the spread of AIDS in Brazil was perceived through its peculiar lens (Daniel, 1985; Galvão, 1985; Trevisan, 1986; see also Chapters 2 and 4 in this volume).[1]

Countering this image with a more empirically grounded understanding of the epidemiology of AIDS in Brazil would prove to be a particularly difficult task for a number of different reasons. On the one hand, access to adequate medical care is often limited, particularly in rural areas as well as among the poorer sectors of more heavily urbanized areas in Brazil, and even where modern medical facilities are available, the complicated symptomatology of HIV infection and AIDS has often made accurate diagnosis notoriously difficult. On the other hand, the weight of prejudice and discrimination has frequently caused both patients and doctors to resist reporting AIDS cases, and even after 1986, when notifying public health officials of cases of AIDS became compulsory, it is likely that the stigma of the disease itself has continued to cause a significant degree of underreporting (ABIA, 1988a, 1988b; Panos Institute, 1988). Even in the light of these problems, however,

Table 1. Cases of AIDS and Number of Deaths by Year, 1980–1992

Year	Number of cases	Number of deaths
1980	1	1
1981	—	—
1982	7	5
1983	32	27
1984	123	103
1985	503	362
1986	987	671
1987	2,284	1,340
1988	3,812	2,065
1989	5,000	2,390
1990	6,535	2,865
1991	7,492	2,610
1992*	1,679	434
Total	28,455	12,873

Note: *Preliminary data through June 1992.
Source: Ministério da Saúde, 1992.

state health organizations in Rio de Janeiro and São Paulo have been registering cases since 1984, and statistics compiled by the Ministry of Health in Brasília have offered at least some sense of an epidemiological reality that diverges sharply from the view of AIDS that has been constructed in the popular imagination (see Tables 1–5).

What is perhaps most striking about the epidemiological picture that has emerged since 1986 is the diversity that it seems to represent in the face of the relatively uniform vision of the epidemic (and of those perceived to be affected) built up in popular culture. By the beginning of 1992, while the highest number of reported cases could still be found in heavily urbanized areas such as the states of São Paulo (17,155 cases, with an incidence rate of 59.2 per 100,000 inhabitants) and Rio de Janeiro (4386 cases, with an incidence rate of 35.0 per 100,000 inhabitants), the spread of the epidemic had already reached every region of the country (see Table 2; on the spread of HIV/AIDS in rural Brazil, see Flowers, 1988).

No less striking, while the sexual transmission of HIV has continued to constitute the single most significant factor in the spread of HIV infection (accounting for 17,392 cases, or 61.1 per cent of the total number of reported cases), only 8749, or 30.7 per cent of the total number of AIDS cases in Brazil were in fact listed as homosexual males. Another 4385 cases, or 15.4 per cent of the national total, were classified as bisexual males, while 4258, or 15.0 per cent of the total number of cases, were linked to heterosexual transmission (see Table 3; Ministério da Saúde, 1992).

*Table 2. Number of Cases and Cases per Million by Region and States or Territories (Unidades Federadas), 1980–1992 ***

REGION/ States and Territories	Number	Cases per 100,000
BRAZIL	**28,455**	**21.4**
NORTH	**280**	**3.5**
Rondônia	16	2.3
Acre	20	5.8
Amazonas	62	3.7
Roraima	27	27.0
Pará	137	3.4
Amapá	8	3.8
Tocantins	10	1.1
NORTHEAST	**2,106**	**5.5**
Maranhão	154	3.4
Piauí	78	3.3
Ceará	318	5.5
Rio Grande do Norte	127	6.1
Paraíba	97	3.3
Pernambuco	572	8.6
Alagoas	108	4.9
Sergipe	69	5.3
Bahia	583	5.5
SOUTHEAST	**22,598**	**51.6**
Minas Gerais	819	5.7
Espírito Santo	238	10.6
Rio de Janeiro	4,386	35.0
São Paulo	17,155	59.2
SOUTH	**2,474**	**12.1**
Paraná	659	8.2
Santa Catarina	481	12.0
Rio Grande do Sul	1,334	15.9
CENTRAL-WEST	**997**	**17.0**
Goiás	246	5.6
Mato Grosso	170	11.9
Mato Grosso do Sul	246	15.7
Distrito Federal	335	22.0

Note: *Through June 1992.
Source: Ministério da Saúde, 1992.

The rapid transition from predominantly homosexual and bisexual transmission to rapidly increasing heterosexual transmission after the first decade becomes even more striking when reported cases of AIDS are viewed across time. While homosexual males accounted for 46.7 per cent, and bisexual males for 22.1 per cent, heterosexual men and women accounted for only 4.9 per cent of the national total between 1980 and 1986. During 1991, on the other hand, cases reported among homosexual men had fallen to 22.9 per cent and cases among bisexual

Table 3. Number and Percentage of Cases of AIDS According to Category of
Transmission and Sex, 1980–1992 *

Category of transmission	Males Number	%	Females Number	%	Total Number	%
Sexual transmission	**15,997**	**64.3**	**1,395**	**39.0**	**17,392**	**61.1**
Homosexual contact	8,749	35.2	—	—	8,749	30.7
Bisexual contact	4,385	17.6	—	—	4,385	15.4
Heterosexual contact	2,863	11.5	1,395	39.0	4,258	15.0
Blood transmission	**6,141**	**24.7**	**1,580**	**44.2**	**7,721**	**27.1**
IV drug use	4,813	19.3	1,073	30.0	5,886	20.7
Transfusion	750	3.0	507	14.2	1,257	4.4
Haemophilia	578	2.3	—	—	578	2.0
Perinatal transmission	**277**	**1.1**	**267**	**7.5**	**544**	**1.9**
Undefined or other	**2,466**	**9.9**	**332**	**9.3**	**2,798**	**9.8**
Total	**24,881**	**87.4+**	**3,574**	**12.6+**	**28,202**	**100.0**

Notes: *Through June 1992.
+Proportional distribution by sex. Male/Female Ratio: 7/1.
Source: Ministério de Saúde, 1992.

men had dropped to 11.1 per cent, while cases reported among heterosexual men and women had risen to 20.1 per cent of the national total
(see Table 4).

Finally, even though cases of blood transmission have rarely received the attention in either the media or the popular imagination that
has been given to the sexual (and especially homosexual) transmission
of HIV in Brazil, the spread of HIV through contact with blood has
continued to be an important source of transmission throughout the
past decade. While people with haemophilia and the recipients of blood
and blood products were especially vulnerable in the early years of the
AIDS epidemic in Brazil, accounting for 7.5 per cent of the cases reported between 1980 and 1986, injecting drug users have increasingly
become a focus for HIV transmission as the epidemic has progressed.
People with haemophilia and the recipients of blood and blood products
continue to account for 3.8 per cent of the cases reported in 1991, for
example, and HIV transmission in relation to injecting drug use has
risen dramatically from 2.8 per cent of the total number of cases reported through 1986 to 26.9 per cent of the cases reported during the
course of 1991. With a particularly strong presence in the highly
populated urban centres of the south and southeast, then, HIV transmission in relation to needle sharing and injecting drug use has taken
shape in the early 1990s as second only to heterosexual contact as the
most rapidly expanding mode of HIV transmission in the country as
a whole (see Table 4).

Table 4. Percentage of Cases by Category of Transmission and Year in Individuals 15 Years or Older.

Category of transmission	1980–86	1987	1988	1989	1990	1991	1992	1980–92
Homosexual	46.7	38.0	33.2	30.4	26.1	22.9	23.5	28.8
Bisexual	22.1	16.4	14.5	13.7	11.3	11.1	12.5	14.2
Heterosexual	4.9	7.5	11.0	14.3	17.2	20.1	23.3	16.5
IV drug use	2.8	11.1	17.4	19.5	23.9	26.9	24.3	20.8
Transfusion	3.9	7.2	5.3	4.3	3.3	2.9	2.6	3.9
Haemophilia	3.6	2.3	2.0	1.5	1.1	0.9	0.7	1.4

Note: *Through June 1992.
Source: Ministério da Saúde, 1992.

Table 5. Number of Cases by Sex, Year of Diagnosis, and Male/Female Ratio, Brazil, 1980–1991

Year of diagnosis	Male	Female	Ratio M/F
1980	1	—	1/—
1981	—	—	—
1982	7	—	7/—
1983	31	1	31/1
1984	122	1	122/1
1985	486	17	29/1
1986	930	57	16/1
1987	2,070	214	10/1
1988	3,327	485	7/1
1989	4,419	581	8/1
1990	5,752	783	7/1
1991	6,337	1,155	5/1
Total	23,482	3,294	7/1

Note: *Through 1 April 1989.
Source: Ministério de Saúde, 1992.

The picture that emerges from the epidemiological data currently available is thus far more complex and varied than the popular image of the AIDS epidemic in Brazil might suggest. Indeed, in spite of gaps and distortions that surely exist in available epidemiological data (see Chapters 2 and 4 in this volume; see also Bastos, 1991), it is clear that the shape of AIDS in Brazil has continued to change in a number of significant ways over the past decade. Perhaps most dramatically, what once appeared to be a disease primarily of homosexual men has rapidly come to have an impact upon a much larger population: the male/female ratio in reported cases of 122/1 in 1984 had fallen to 5/1 by 1991 (see Table 5). While the continued importance of male homosexual practices in the spread of HIV infection in Brazil can hardly be denied, given the rapid increase of both heterosexual transmission and HIV infection in relation to injecting drug use, it is equally impossible to characterize AIDS in Brazil solely along these lines.

At the same time, and clearly in relation to such shifts in HIV transmission, the social and economic profile of the epidemic has rapidly changed, increasingly affecting the poorest sectors of Brazilian society — unquestionably the greatest mass of what is an overwhelmingly poor nation. Far from a disease limited to the most elite, well-to-do sectors of Brazilian society, the epidemic has cut across class and status boundaries, taking its greatest toll on members of the lower-middle and lower classes (see Guimarães *et al.*, 1988). This hardly seems surprising, of course, in a society that has traditionally failed to resolve even the most basic health problems of the poor — in which the widespread existence of homelessness, children earning their living in the streets, and both female and male prostitution for survival are common facts of daily life. Increasingly, it would appear that regardless of the stereotypes and prejudices ingrained in the popular view of AIDS in Brazil, the reality of the epidemic is the reality of Brazilian society as a whole. In many ways, therefore, the face of AIDS in Brazil is the face of Brazil itself (ABIA, 1988b).[2]

The Social and Cultural Contexts of HIV Infection

If the picture that has gradually begun to emerge of the AIDS epidemic in Brazil differs in a number of significant ways from the stereotypes that have marked the popular discussion of the disease, it has offered only limited insight into the social conditions that have actually structured the development of the epidemic. To understand more fully not only the spread of the disease, but also the ways in which Brazilian society has responded to it, we must ultimately turn to a wider social and cultural context — in particular, to the beliefs and practices that structure sexual interactions or contacts, the exchange of blood and blood products, and the use of injecting drugs. If, in Brazil as in other societies, it is through such behaviours that the transmission of HIV has taken place, the ways in which such behaviours take shape are anything but random, and understanding the specific character and development of AIDS in Brazil depends on some understanding of the ways in which such practices are socially and culturally constituted (ABIA, 1988a, 1988b; Chapter 4 in this volume).

Nowhere is this more evident than in the case of sexuality. While the discussion of AIDS in Brazil has been carried out largely in terms of categories such as '*homossexualidade*' ('homosexuality'), '*bissexualidade*' ('bisexuality') and '*heterossexualidade*' ('heterosexuality'), these categories are highly problematic within the context of Brazilian sexual culture. While they are the most salient classifications structuring the sexual universe in the United States and perhaps much of Western Europe, they are actually quite recent importations in Brazil. They certainly do exist in Brazilian culture, particularly in the discourse of the medical sciences, but they are not necessarily the categories that most Brazilians use to think about the nature of sexual reality. On the contrary, their impact has generally been limited to a relatively small segment of Brazilian society: an educated elite drawn principally from the middle and upper classes in the most modern urban areas (Fry, 1982; Fry and MacRae, 1983; Parker, 1989, 1991, Chapter 4 in this volume).

Traditionally, categories such as *homossexualidade* and *heterossexualidade* have been far less significant within the ideological structure of Brazilian sexual culture than what we might describe as notions of *'atividade'* ('activity') and *'passividade'* ('passivity'). Particularly among males from the popular sectors of Brazilian society, the so-called 'active' partners in same-sex interactions, for example, do not necessarily consider themselves to be either *'homossexual'* ('homosexual') or *'bissexual'* ('bisexual') — designations which are more commonly reserved, if they are used at all, for the perceived 'passive' partners in these interactions. While a heavy stigma has always been attached to male passivity (see Misse, 1981), activity in occasional same-sex sexual relations has been relatively unproblematic.[3] Indeed, there would even seem to be a certain possibility for the negotiation of active and passive sexual performances in same-sex interactions, and same-sex sexual relations do not, by any means, preclude sexual interactions with the opposite sex predicated on the assumption of male activity and female passivity. In short, while sexual roles (like partners) may vary, they tend to be far more significant than sexual object choice in the construction of sexual identity (Fry, 1982; Fry and MacRae, 1983; Parker, 1989, 1991, Chapter 4 in this volume; Perlongher, 1987a).

A product of this particular configuration of the sexual universe, then, has been a certain fluidity in the construction of sexual relationships in Brazil. What we might describe as a sexual subculture focused on same-sex interactions has been a part of Brazilian urban life since at least the early part of the twentieth century, and has become increasingly visible over the course of the past three decades (Parker, 1989; Perlongher, 1987b; Trevisan, 1986). The boundaries of this subculture have been relatively flexible, however, and it has been organized less around a shared *'identidade homossexual'* ('homosexual identity') than around a set of quite diverse same-sex desires and practices (see Chapter 4 in this volume). What might be described (even if with a certain degree of exaggeration) as the relative uniformity of the gay subculture in the United States, for example, is altogether absent in Brazil, where a plurality of classifications and identities come together without ever forming a single, clearly defined social group.

This configuration has been particularly important in Brazil, of course, with the emergence of the HIV/AIDS epidemic. The existence of this distinct sexual subculture has at once provided a space for the spread of the epidemic, while at the same time giving it its unique character and directionality: its early emergence among males involved in same-sex relations along with its rapid development among males involved in relations with both the same and the opposite sexes. At the same time the particular form of this subculture has also influenced the ways in which Brazilian society has responded to it. Indeed, the general lack of a clearly defined community with its own institutional structure and self-identified constituency has severely limited the ability of the population that has experienced the greatest risk of HIV infection both to act on its own behalf as well as to exert political pressure for action on the part of the state. The kinds of education and information campaigns mounted by gay groups in the United States or the countries of Western Europe, along with the important activities of voluntary organizations committed to the care and treatment of people with HIV/AIDS, have been almost unknown in Brazil, and the pressure politics necessary to counteract government inactivity in these other countries have been largely impossible in a setting where gay political groups are both very limited and factionalized (see Parker, 1989, 1993).

Just as the social construction of the sexual universe has left its own distinct mark on the development of AIDS in Brazil, the specific practices that have determined the flow of blood have also shaped the development of the epidemic and the ways in which Brazilian society has been able to respond to it (ABIA, 1988a, 1988b; Ramos, 1988). The lack of effective regulation and control over the supply of blood is a longstanding problem in Brazil. In part, of course, this lack of an effective regulatory system is the result of certain fairly easily understandable limitations in the more general public health system — limitations which are themselves linked to the complicated problems of economic development. At the same time, however, the problem can also be tied to a culturally constituted ideological system in which blood donation is valued not as a humanitarian act but as a source of income (ABIA, 1988b; Castro *et al.*, 1987). As much as 70 per cent of the blood that is collected and processed in the state of Rio de Janeiro, for example, is in the hands of private commercial organizations using paid blood donors (Padilha, 1988). Blood donation has thus traditionally been the province of the poorest sectors of Brazilian society (the same sectors, of course, that have the least access to adequate medical care), and an entire class of 'professional blood donors' who sell their blood in order to meet the most minimal conditions of material existence has become an integral part of the Brazilian blood market (ABIA, 1988b; Castro *et al.*, 1987).

The extensive commercialization of the blood supply, together with a lack of rigour in government regulation of the blood industry in Brazil, has traditionally led to high incidence of transfusion-associated infectious diseases such as syphilis, hepatitis and Chagas' disease (Padilha, 1988). It is estimated, for example, that as many as

20,000 new cases of Chagas' disease are caused each year in Brazil by transfusions of infected blood (ABIA, 1988b). The already significant problems associated with the blood supply have only been accentuated by the emergence of AIDS. In Rio de Janeiro, for example, one study of 100 homeless people found that 70 per cent were professional blood donors — and that 7 per cent were HIV positive (Carvalho *et al.*, 1987). In the mid-1980s one of every five cases of AIDS reported in Rio was due to contaminated blood (ABIA, 1988b).

Although the gravity of this situation has led to government decrees aimed at ensuring that blood banks test for HIV, in practice the cost of testing has meant that such regulations have been widely ignored. In contrast to the United States and Western Europe, the Brazilian government seems to have been relatively powerless to enforce its own decrees and prevent their circumvention, and precisely where the enforcement of regulations related to blood screening has been the most rigorous, as in states such as Rio de Janeiro and São Paulo, it seems to have simultaneously given rise to an entire network of clandestine blood banks run for profit by racketeers who fiercely resist government regulation. In Rio de Janeiro alone, while nearly a dozen clandestine blood banks were shut down in 1988, the director of the state health inspection unit estimated that more than thirty others may have escaped detection (*San Francisco Chronicle*, 1988). As in the case of the population involved in same-sex sexual practices, there exists little in the way of organized political pressure groups capable of pushing for more effective control of the blood supply. Associations representing people with haemophilia have been active, and there seems to be far greater public sympathy for the plight of people with HIV/AIDS infected through blood transfusions (who are frequently portrayed as 'innocent victims' in contrast to individuals infected through their own wilful sexual behaviours), but their ability to influence the political process in any significant way has been limited at best, and their impact has probably been no greater than that of the few gay liberation organizations that have focused on AIDS as a social and political issue.[4]

Finally, although injecting drug use lagged behind other modes of transmission during the early years of the AIDS epidemic in Brazil, it has recently become one the most rapidly expanding modes of HIV transmission, and currently accounts for more than 20 per cent of the total number of cases reported in the country as a whole (see Table 3). Indeed, during 1991 HIV transmission associated with injecting drug use surpassed male homosexual contact as the most frequently reported mode of transmission, accounting for 26.9 per cent of the reported cases of AIDS (see Table 4), and in some areas, such as parts of the state of São Paulo, this percentage is significantly higher, and has been especially difficult to confront.

If such trends seem to mirror similar tendencies in the United States and parts of Western Europe, however, it is important to remember that even here a range of highly specific social, cultural, economic and political factors have shaped the changing epidemiology of HIV/AIDS in relation to injecting drug use in Brazil. It is impossible, for example, to separate the rapid increase in HIV infection through injecting drug use in Brazil from the perhaps unintended, and certainly unforeseen, impact of American foreign policy and drug enforcement activities in South America. It is possible to trace, year by year and along highly specific geographic routes, the spread of HIV infection among injecting drug users in Brazil during the late 1980s in relation to a range of activities aimed at cutting off the flow of cocaine from highland South America (and especially Bolivia) to the US marketplace. As the drug traffic routes out of Bolivia and Columbia were regulated more severely, Brazil's largely unregulated Amazonian borders became increasingly attractive, and its active port system became a convenient route out of South America to the United States, Western Europe and even West Africa (see Mesquita, 1992).

By the late 1980s, then, a swath of drug traffic routes had spread down from the Amazon basin, through São Paulo and on to port cities such as Rio de Janeiro and Santos. As is always the case, drug trafficking functions best with an extensive pool of cheap and largely captive labour, easily controlled by drug addiction itself. In Brazil the implications for HIV infection have been all the more serious because injection has been almost exclusively linked to cocaine, a drug which, unlike heroin, produces a relatively short-lived effect, and thus tends to be reinjected with relative frequency, greatly expanding the risk of rapid HIV transmission when injecting practices are associated with needle sharing.

While the sale of needles is not illegal in Brazil, their price is clearly prohibitive, particularly given the fact that drug injection has become most frequent among the poorest, most marginalized sectors of Brazilian society. The prevention of HIV transmission in relation to injecting drug use has been complicated further still by the fact that drug use has traditionally been treated as a legal, rather than a medical, issue, and that the possibility of prevention activities such as needle exchange programs for injecting drug users has been completely restricted by legal sanctions. Increasingly, then, a subculture of injecting drug use, associated with drug trafficking, and exhibiting high rates of needle sharing as a response to economic and legal restraints, has taken shape in the large urban centres of south and southeast Brazil, and rates of HIV infection among drug users have risen dramatically, virtually guaranteeing that HIV infection in relation to injecting drug use will continue to be a central component of the AIDS epidemic in Brazil throughout the foreseeable future.

Brazil, of course, is an immensely diverse country, and the shape of the AIDS epidemic varies to some degree in different areas — just as AIDS in San Francisco differs in important ways from AIDS in New York, and AIDS in Kinshasa differs from AIDS in rural parts of Zaire. While HIV transmission through injecting drug use remains limited in many parts of the country, for example, it is already extensive in areas such as the city and state of São Paulo. Indeed, it would be more accurate to describe the HIV/AIDS epidemic in Brazil less as a single, unified pattern than as a myriad of epicentres, each with its own peculiar characteristics. Perhaps the most important point, however, is that these multiple, criss-crossing patterns have been shaped by the specific social, cultural, economic and political circumstances of contemporary Brazilian life. As much as the cultural images that AIDS has engendered, the apparently concrete patterns of HIV transmission are themselves constructed (in Brazil as elsewhere). They are moulded by forces that are at once local and global, reflecting, at one and the same time, the relatively fluid and open-ended nature of sexual contacts, particularly among males in Brazilian society, as well as the blatant commercialization of blood and blood products, and even the unwitting consequences of distant decisions and geopolitical concerns shaping international drug enforcement policies.

The Politics of AIDS in Brazil

Just as specific social and cultural contexts have so significantly structured the changing shape of HIV infection and AIDS in Brazil, these same forces have simultaneously conditioned the ways in which Brazilian society has responded to the epidemic. As in every society, this response has been complicated and difficult, uncovering, like the epidemic itself, the hidden tensions of contemporary life — the unexamined and unrecognized fissures of the social landscape. In Brazil it has been complicated further by yet another set of circumstances: by a specific historical moment, and, in particular, a complicated set of social and political transformations that have profoundly influenced the ways in which Brazilian society has responded to the AIDS epidemic. Perhaps even more than the factors that we have examined thus far — or, at the very least, interacting with them — it is this historical context that has shaped what we might describe as the politics of AIDS in Brazil.

It is absolutely crucial to remember that the emergence of the AIDS epidemic in Brazil between 1982 and 1984 coincided almost completely with the development of a social, political and economic crisis that has been accurately described as probably the worst in Brazilian history (ABIA, 1988b). The first cases of AIDS were reported in 1982 and 1983, during the last of five military governments that had ruled the country since the coup of 1964, and the continued spread of the epidemic has been played out against the backdrop of the country's tentative, and at times tenuous, return to civilian rule. At the same time the economic crisis, linked to Brazil's immense foreign debt and the politics of both international lending and economic dependency, has generally accentuated already existing problems in the structure of the country's public health system while simultaneously limiting the government's ability to respond to the problems posed by a new epidemic disease. For better or for worse, the politics of AIDS in Brazil has been played out in relation to this wider historical and economic context (ABIA, 1988b).

Perhaps the most significant consequence of this has been the widely felt sense, on the part of the Brazilian people, that neither individual citizens nor non-government organizations are truly capable of significantly influencing the political process. This sense of a certain political impotence was itself the product of twenty years of authoritarian rule, in which civil liberties and the rights of citizens were widely disregarded, followed by what might be described as a kind of collapse of hope in relation to the return to civilian government. The late 1970s and the early 1980s — a period described by the military rulers themselves as one of '*abertura*' or 'opening' in preparation for a return to civilian rule — were characterized by extensive social and political action. Feminism, the ecology movement and the Black movement all flourished in Brazil during this period of gradual liberalization, as did a number of gay liberation groups, and there was considerable optimism concerning the political future of the country. Much of this political energy focused, in 1983 and 1984, on the campaign for '*Diretas Já*': a campaign for the direct election, by popular vote, of Brazil's first civilian president in more than two decades. While it brought large segments of the population into the streets for demonstrations across the country, however, this campaign for direct elections was ultimately a failure, as the last military government refused to give up its plan for a more gradual return of power to civilian society.

It is difficult to describe, particularly for readers unfamiliar with the psychological effects of life under authoritarian rule, the impact that the failure of the campaign for direct elections had on Brazilian political life. So much energy had been focused on this question that its negative resolution created a kind of void or vacuum in public life, and large segments of the population watched the activities of the new republican government with a high degree of scepticism. A sense of optimism began to surface once again in 1986, when the new administration launched the '*Plano Cruzado*', an economic plan aimed at ending Brazil's spiraling inflation and predicated on the active involvement of the civilian population as watchdogs charged with regulating merchants to ensure compliance with price controls. Once again, however, the ultimate failure of the initiative, the declaration of a moratorium on foreign debt payments, and the return to an inflationary economy transformed the optimism of 1986 into an increasingly bleak pessimism in 1987 and 1988, as members of the politically influential middle class began to give up hope and a widespread exodus to live and work abroad became part of modern Brazilian life.

While these developments seem far removed from the development of the AIDS epidemic, they are intimately tied up with it, as they have profoundly influenced the political climate that has in turn determined AIDS policy. On the one hand, the tension between holdovers of authoritarianism and hopes for democracy seems to have reproduced itself in AIDS-related policies, while the economic crisis has further complicated the problem of AIDS funding by severely limiting the available resources for all public health initiatives, and thus making the competition for health-related spending all the more extreme. The general sense of despair in civil society concerning the impact that both individuals and groups can have in influencing the political process has, in turn, accentuated the already acute absence of voluntary groups with clearly identified constituencies at risk for the transmission of AIDS, and has limited the level of participation in organizations aimed at influencing AIDS-related public policy. While the role of the state has thus emerged as fundamental to meeting the problems associated with AIDS in Brazil, a whole range of forces seems to have combined to limit the influence that civil society has been able to exert in shaping the policies and activities of the state.

The result of these various circumstances has been an at times frightening climate of prejudice and discrimination, on the one hand, linked to delays in government action and the sometimes directionless development of public policy, on the other hand. A general lack of information and, perhaps even worse, misinformation have resulted in a whole catalogue of individual cruelties, as persons assumed (correctly or incorrectly) to be infected with HIV have quite literally been run out of town or suffered threats of physical violence (see, for example, *Veja*, 1985b; *Isto é Senhor*, 1988). Perhaps even more worrying, precisely those individuals and institutions that might be expected to be leaders in AIDS awareness have often been anything but, as both individual doctors as well as leading hospitals have often refused to treat AIDS patients (see *Veja*, 1985a, 1987, 1988; Mott, 1987; Trevisan, 1986), while other medical experts have disseminated inflammatory, alarmist and sometimes blatantly untrue information that has done little more than incite prejudices against those affected by the epidemic (see Mott, 1987; Perlongher, 1987a; Trevisan, 1986). The vestiges of an institutionalized authoritarianism have at times been frighteningly evident in the persecution of perceived risk groups such as male homosexuals, female prostitutes and transvestites, who have frequently been the victims of police violence legitimized and justified as AIDS prevention activities (*New York Times*, 1987b; Perlongher, 1987b; see also Chapter 3 in this volume).

This general climate must be linked, of course, to a series of delays in the development of a national AIDS policy. As in so many other nations, even after the epidemic began to become statistically significant, the Brazilian government was slow to take action. Inactivity was justified, at first, by the immensity of Brazil's other unresolved public health problems — a few hundred cases of AIDS seemed relatively inconsequential in comparison to thousands of cases of Chagas' disease, malaria, tuberculosis, meningitis and the like (*New York Times*, 1985; Panos Institute, 1988). In addition, the severe financial strains of Brazil's extended economic crisis have consistently been cited as unavoidable pressures limiting the availability of funding for basic research, educational programs and the care and treatment of AIDS patients (*Jornal do Brasil*, 1986).

As the numbers began to mount, the potential impact of the epidemic became more evident, and international attention began to focus on government inactivity in Brazil. The Ministry of Health finally began to take action (*Newsweek*, 1987; *New York Times*, 1986, 1987b; Panos Institute, 1988). Perhaps most significantly, in May 1985 a government *Portaria* or 'Executive Order' called for the establishment of a *Programa Nacional de DST/AIDS* (National STD/AIDS Program) to be elaborated by a new *Divisão Nacional de Controle de Doenças Sexualmente Transmissíveis e SIDA-AIDS* (National Division for the Control of Sexually Transmitted Diseases and SIDA-AIDS) within the Ministry of Health; and this newly formed unit began work on elaborating an extensive five-year plan aimed at directing Brazil's response to the epidemic between 1988 and 1992 (see Ministério de Saúde, 1987; see also Rodrigues, 1988b).

Even following the formation of a new institutional structure aimed at responding to the epidemic, however, it was only at the end of 1986 that the Minister of Health signed a further order mandating compulsory notification of AIDS cases and making it possible to begin to track the epidemic nationally, and even after this it has been largely impossible to ensure full compliance on the part of doctors who often follow their patients' wishes in failing to record the AIDS diagnosis (ABIA, 1988b; Panos Institute, 1988). In May 1987, in turn, the Ministry of Health ordered the screening of blood donations, but the lack of both legal sanctions and an official regulatory apparatus has made it impossible to enforce screening procedures (*New York Times*, 1987a).[5] Finally, while education and information have been seen as the key to reducing the spread of the epidemic, it has only been in 1987 and 1988 that a large-scale educational program began to be implemented and that the mass media began to be used as an integral part of the educational process (*New York Times*, 1987b; *Visão*, 1987). Even here, the explicit nature of the information presented has drawn the criticism of conservative forces such as the Roman Catholic Church, and it has sometimes been necessary to revise educational campaigns not to increase their effectiveness, but to avoid offending moral sensibilities (*New York Times*, 1987b).[6]

Throughout the past decade the fight against AIDS in Brazil has been carried out in the face of a continued lack of adequate funding for even the most basic programs. Virtually all major AIDS-related research in Brazil has had to rely on funding and expertise from external sources such as the Pan American Health Organization, the Centers for Disease Control and the National Institutes for Health in the United States — and, as a result, has also had to respond to a research agenda determined in the vastly different social setting of North America.[7] In September 1988, as the spread of the epidemic continued to increase by nearly 100 per cent per year, the federal government announced a reduction of 30 per cent in AIDS funding, leaving the Ministry of Health's National AIDS Program without sufficient funds for basic medicines and blood testing supplies (*Jornal do Brasil*, 1988). While help from private foundations and the international health community has increasingly been made available (and will need to be expanded in the future), a basic commitment to combatting the epidemic has yet to emerge from the government in Brasília; and the Ministry of Health's own AIDS team has been left alarmingly understaffed and underfunded (*Jornal do Brasil*, 1988; *O Globo*, 1988).[8]

At the same time that the history of AIDS had been marked by discrimination, neglect and official inactivity. However, in Brazil, as in so many other countries, a critical response to this record has gradually begun to emerge, and is itself perhaps the other side of the increasingly widespread lack of confidence in the established institutions of Brazilian society. Indeed, to a large extent this response seems to have depended on a certain kind of disgust in the face of institutional inactivity, and a sense that nothing will be done if individual citizens fail to take matters into their own hands. In a number of fairly limited instances it has emerged from already existing organizations in the gay liberation movement, which have become increasingly active in distributing educational and informational materials (interestingly, the groups with the greatest sense of the diversity of Brazilian sexual and homosexual culture seem to have been the most active, while those more fully committed to Western European and North American models have generally been less likely to focus on AIDS education).

Perhaps even more commonly, however, the rise of AIDS activism has taken shape not within already existing organizations originally founded in relation to other issues, but through the formation of new organizations specifically in response to the many complicated problems raised by the epidemic. Since late 1985, when government initiatives were still in their infancy, these new AIDS organizations have increasingly constituted not only the most important critics of government inertia, but often, as well, the leaders in AIDS education, in the defence of civil liberties for people with AIDS, and even in the provision of basic care and treatment services for AIDS patients.

Already, the early results of such activities offer at least some reason for a certain degree of optimism. The pressure applied by such organizations has increasingly brought a more reasoned and reasonable consideration of AIDS into the media, and has gradually begun to shake the largely erroneous popular stereotype of the disease and its perceived victims. In addition, the efforts of AIDS activists seem to have pushed the medical/scientific establishment and the Ministry of Health in the direction of a greater sensitivity in relation to both the nuances of Brazilian sexual culture and the need for an understanding of social diversity in relation to AIDS. Leading NGO representatives have been included, for example, along with medical doctors, scientists and public health officials in the formation of the Ministry of Health's *Comissão Nacional de Controle de AIDS* (National AIDS Commission). While there is obviously much to be done in a situation that is becoming more and more critical with each passing day, the gradual emergence of a critical dialogue between the state and voluntary sectors of Brazilian society offers the possibility, perhaps for the first time, of forging policy initiatives that will truly respond to the reality of the AIDS epidemic in Brazil.

Conclusion

Precisely because AIDS is a disease that is spread through socially determined practices, the shape that it takes in any given setting is as much a product of social and cultural structures as it is the result of biological factors. By extension, just as a specific set of social and cultural circumstances shapes the spread of AIDS, it also conditions the ways in which particular societies respond to it — the ways in which they define or interpret the disease, the reactions they have in relation to those affected by it, the steps they take to prevent it and so on. While the specific case of AIDS in Brazil has drawn somewhat less attention than a number of other cases, it is nonetheless instructive. Precisely because it presents a number of significant differences when compared with other, better known patterns, it perhaps offers the chance, at least partially, to rethink, within a comparative framework, our understanding not only of the disease itself, but also of its profound social consequences elsewhere in the world.

International epidemiologists have tended to focus on two major patterns of HIV transmission. The first of these patterns places central emphasis on transmission principally through male homosexual relations and injecting drug use, and has been identified in the countries of Western Europe, Australia, New Zealand and most of North and South America. The second places emphasis on transmission principally through heterosexual relations and transfusions with contaminated blood, and has been identified in the countries of Africa as well as in a number of the nations of the Caribbean (Piot *et al.*, 1988; Quinn *et al.*, 1986). Although Brazil has typically been included as another example of the first of these patterns (see Piot *et al.*, 1988), a closer inspection of the details of the Brazilian case suggests a number of important differences when compared with both of these patterns or models of HIV transmission (see also Chapters 2 and 4 in this volume).

On the one hand, as in the United States and Western Europe, a high percentage of the AIDS cases thus far reported in Brazil has been linked to male homosexual contacts. Yet cases of AIDS linked to bisexual contacts have also been unusually common, and heterosexual transmission has become increasingly significant with each passing year, emerging, by the end of the first decade of the epidemic, as the most rapidly expanding mode of HIV transmission in the country as a whole. On the other hand, as in the developing countries of Africa and the Caribbean, AIDS cases linked to transfusion with contaminated blood have been relatively common, and continue to be recorded with disconcerting frequency. At the same time, however, HIV infection in relation to injecting drug use (which seems to be almost unknown in most of Africa) has increased rapidly in recent years, dominating the epidemiological profile in at least some parts of the country.

Understanding these complex and changing patterns (which seem to combine elements that have been seen as distinct in the epidemiology of AIDS in other parts of the world), in turn, requires some understanding of the specific details of Brazilian social life — in particular, its relatively open-ended configuration of the sexual universe combined with the uncontrolled commercialization of the exchange of blood and blood products and its rapidly expanding injecting drug using subculture. Taken together, these social and cultural factors simultaneously distinguish the Brazilian case from better known examples in North America or central Africa, while at the same time perhaps linking it to any number of other Latin American, and even some Asian, societies. Indeed, they suggest that they very notion of overriding patterns characterizing the global epidemiology of AIDS may well be giving way with the passage of time — and that such patterns, to the extent that they do exist, may often threaten to obscure the particularities of HIV transmission in specific settings.

The specificity of such differences is just as important in turning from the spread and development of the epidemic itself to the ways in which society has responded to it. The same kinds of social factors that condition the transmission of HIV also influence the ways in which different societies seek to confront it. The case of Brazil is in a number of ways significantly different from those of the major Anglo-American or Western European nations, on the one hand, and the countries of central Africa and the Caribbean, on the other hand. While male homosexual and bisexual sexual contacts have accounted for a particularly high percentage of the reported cases of HIV/AIDS in Brazil, the lack of a gay community organized along the lines of the gay community in the countries of the fully developed and industrialized West has clearly had a significant impact on the initial response of Brazilian society in the face of the epidemic, and continues to be a significant factor in the particular way in which the politics of AIDS has developed in contemporary Brazilian life. And while the contamination of blood and blood products has been important in Brazil, unlike many of the other countries in the developing world, this has been less the result of economic underdevelopment itself — i.e., an absolute lack of necessary resources — than the result of a particular set of social and political forces that has simultaneously transformed blood into a market commodity while undercutting efforts that might regulate or inhibit the highest available profit margin. Ironically, many of these same market forces have simultaneously contributed to the rapid expansion of injecting drug use in Brazil (precisely as they have sought to respond to the regulation of drug use in other parts of the world), leaving Brazilian society particularly vulnerable to the rapid influx of new, and only poorly understood, behaviours associated with perhaps the most potentially explosive dimension of the epidemic.

These various factors, in turn, must be linked to the specificity of a particular historical moment — to Brazil's tentative transition from an authoritarian military government to a civilian democracy facing a set of profoundly difficult social and economic problems. While this transition has taken place with what might be described as relative stability when compared with some of the countries (for example, Uganda or Haiti) where the increase of HIV transmission has been particularly severe, it might simultaneously appear to be disjointed and uneasy at best when compared with the representative democracies of any number of other nations (Australia, France, the United States and so on) faced with the problems raised by the epidemic. As in so many other developing nations, the transition from authoritarian dictatorship to tentative democracy has been played out, as well, in the midst of an economic crisis created by the politics of economic dependency. While the resources available for the fight against AIDS have in no way been as limited as those available in most African or Caribbean nations, their scarcity has nonetheless created a distinct set of pressures that is qualitatively different from that found in the wealthier nations of the fully industrialized West — a set of pressures that has unavoidably shaped the response to the epidemic in a number of highly specific ways. Along with the wider social and cultural context, then, this historical situation has played a fundamental role in determining both the form of the HIV/AIDS epidemic in Brazil and the ways in which Brazilian society has responded to it.

Ultimately, then, the record of the first decade of the AIDS epidemic in Brazil must be read against the background of a complex set of social, cultural, political and economic circumstances. If the face of AIDS is the face of Brazilian society, then the social history of the epidemic is also the history of Brazil itself. As any number of the activist groups that have begun to organize around AIDS in Brazil have themselves demonstrated, critically analyzing this history, and the specific circumstances that have produced it, is perhaps the first step toward inventing a more effective response in the future. This is no less true as we turn from a single case to the wider context of the international pandemic: understanding the specific forces that have shaped the history of AIDS in different societies, and situating these societies in a comparative framework, are necessarily the first steps in seeking to build a more effective global response to the epidemic in the future. It is among the most significant contributions (and, by extension, should be seen as among the most pressing projects) that social analysis can make in responding to what can quite accurately be described as among the most serious problems currently facing the international community.

Notes

1 Even some Ministers of Health have had a role to play in constructing this image, characterizing AIDS, even in the late 1980s, as a 'disease of the elite', and apparently justifying the withholding of resources for diagnosis, treatment and prevention on the grounds that the middle and upper classes can afford the expense of such services (*Folha de São Paulo*, 1988a).

2 Given the general lack of data on the social background or class standing of people with HIV/AIDS in Brazil, it is difficult to develop an empirically-based picture of the epidemic in the country as a whole (*Folha de São Paulo*, 1988a). Interviews with AIDS researchers and physicians throughout the country confirm the results of limited studies such as Guimarães *et al.* (1988) and Grangeiro (1992) in pointing to the current cross-class dimensions of the epidemic. Since many of the very earliest cases of AIDS in Brazil were recorded among relatively well-to-do individuals who frequently spent extensive time travelling or living abroad, however, it would seem (even if in only impressionistic terms) that the AIDS epidemic in Brazil, as in nations such as the United States and France, has been adrift socially downwards. This impression is confirmed, as well, by the recent increase in cases of AIDS among injecting drug users, who tend to be members of the poorer sectors of Brazilian society.

3 The use of terms 'active' and 'passive' from popular Brazilian Portuguese has been intentionally maintained here, as opposed to more neutral or social scientific terminology such as 'insertive' and 'receptive', in order to emphasize the hierarchical distinctions implicit in popular culture. It is perhaps worth noting that although homosexuality is not a legal offence in Brazil, police oppression or harassment of perceived homosexuals frequently occurs. Such harassment is predicated not on legitimate legal

constraints, however, but on popular prejudices — in particular, on stigmas related to male effeminacy or passivity.

4 Associations of people with haemophilia have existed for some decades, both on the national level as well as in each different state. Traditionally, however, they have tended to serve largely as self-help organizations. With the emergence of AIDS, this general orientation has begun to give way to an increasing politicization, and haemophilia associations have been heavily involved in seeking to shape more effective policies for the regulation of the blood supply. Even though a relatively high degree of public sympathy exists for the plight of people with haemophilia in the face of AIDS, however, their relatively limited numbers also limit their potential influence in a political system that rarely responds to the interests of groups that exert no special economic power.

5 Brazil's new Constitution, which went into effect in October 1988, technically outlaws the commercial sale of blood and blood products. The Brazilian Congress has passed a number of laws to enforce the Constitution, but it remains to be seen whether or not the commercialization of blood can be effectively controlled within a public health system that frequently fails to enforce existing legislation.

6 The response of the Catholic Church, and of religious groups in general, to the problems raised by AIDS in Brazil has generally been highly conservative, and at times even reactionary (see Mott, 1985). The internal politics of the Church in Brazil are complicated, however, and there is a strong liberal/left faction. These divisions have been reflected in the response of the Church to the AIDS epidemic, and specific policies have varied widely from region to region (see Regan, 1987). The Ministry of Health has sought to work as closely as possible in collaboration with the Church (see Rodrigues, 1988a), sometimes bending to Church pressure and sometimes managing to secure the cooperation of the Church. In early public service announcements on television, for example, the Ministry of Health was forced to drop the use of the term 'camisinha' — from 'camisinha de Vênus' (literally, 'Venus' little T-shirt'), the popular designation for the condom — due to the opposition of religious leaders; the more explicit language reappeared, however, in later television announcements, without significant comment on the part of Church officials.

7 The role of economic dependency in AIDS research is complicated enough to warrant a study in its own right. In Brazil, at least, it seems to have raised problems on a number of different levels. The focus of research projects sometimes responds to problems that are thus far relatively insignificant in Brazil (but that may be of interest to foreign funding agencies because of their importance in North America or Western Europe), while other questions that may actually prove to be more significant within the Brazilian context are left altogether unstudied. Collaborative work with foreign institutions also raises its own problems — some foreign researchers exhibit a rather remarkable degree of misinformation concerning the

shape of the AIDS epidemic in Brazil, while Brazilian researchers sometimes complain about exploitation in the division of labour established for
collaborative projects.

8 For a fuller discussion of the development of AIDS-related policy in Brazil, and of successive changes in the National AIDS Program in particular,
see Parker, 1993.

Chapter 2

The Bankruptcy of the Models: Myths and Realities of AIDS in Brazil

Herbert Daniel

The AIDS epidemic did not take Brazil by surprise. To the contrary, its coming was announced by many: physicians, scientists, journalists and politicians. The press, more or less following the international news columns, especially those of the United States, had been carrying important items on the subject since 1982. The prevailing mood at the time was one of perplexity tinged with a sense of the exotic.

The first reports drew most of their information from American and European publications, but local stories were also included. A 'scientific' report in *Veja* in July 1982, for example, told of the research of a professor in Bahia who asserted on the basis of his clinical experience that the infection could be traced to the abuse of injectable female hormones and 'infected' silicone by male homosexuals, at a time when, pursuing a theory of infection by a new virus, French scientists were already isolating LAV (later renamed HIV, the human immunodeficiency virus).

Needless to say, ideas of this kind, which proliferated at the time, disappeared soon after, swept away by the cleansing action of common sense. Others came to take their place, however, proving that 'blaming the victim' may be an indelible part of human nature. The press, which fuelled most of the public debates, played up the more striking and enigmatic side of the epidemic, and especially the almost direct association the disease seemed to forge between the twin taboos of sex and death. In its issue of 15 June 1983 *Veja* carried a feature under the title 'O Enigma que Mata' (The Enigma that Kills). AIDS was depicted as a mystery, something beyond the technological capacity of the modern world, with death as its most distinguishing feature.

In Brazil, where gay or homosexual society is less organized than in the United States and Western Europe, the fact that AIDS in these regions affected mostly gay men aroused ambiguous emotions that did little to attract either serious or responsible journalism. By about 1983 all that remained was to expect confirmation of the presence of the disease in Brazil, and the press needed only the name of the first 'victim' to trigger headlines already composed in advance. In 1983 these headlines appeared, as Brazil witnessed its first public case of AIDS. During this year a veritable upsurge of press interest focused on what was then objectively referred to as the 'gay cancer' or 'gay plague'.

This expectation was not merely sensationalist, as there was real concern about the possible impact of the new epidemic. Many alarms were sounded, warnings given, predictions offered, and announcements made. But none of this resulted in preventive action. No measures were set in motion — especially not by the health authorities — to confront an epidemic that no one doubted would arrive in the country.

The fact that 'AIDS' arrived, in a sense, before AIDS itself, resulted in the adoption of an inappropriate ideological model that has guided Brazil's responses to the epidemic up to the present. It is the features of this model that I will discuss here. The principal characteristic of the predominant model of AIDS generated in Brazil, and relied upon by the government and the people, is not that this is a disease of gay man, or of the very poor, but a disease of 'others', of strange and foreign people. There is no logical reason to expect that Brazil would follow the North American epidemiological model, except for incorrect information and cultural colonialism. Because the epidemic 'seemed to have come' from the United States, its model had to be a copy of the 'American model'. As a result, there was no criticism, either of the adequacy of the model and its characteristics or of its mechanical application. An effort to understand this model is an important part of the effort to dispel some of the myths that have contributed to government immobility and brought suffering and despair to many who suffer more from the imposed model of AIDS than from the terrible effects of HIV.

I speak more than anything else from the standpoint of one who lives with AIDS. I have learned to live with a disease that does not conform to the patterning of any formal set of understandings. I know that freeing myself from the model has been essential to my own survival, for it was a struggle against legal death imposed by a view that, in other countries as well as in Brazil, makes the person with AIDS a pariah. Important as this resistance is to the individual, I think it is just as important to society to cast off the model and its preconceptions and attempt to integrate into the community the millions of Brazilians who already have AIDS today. But there are millions more who remain oblivious to the disease because they feel it has no bearing on their daily lives, and they, too, must be protected from it. This stance of solidarity seems to me the best vantage from which to talk about the possible impact of AIDS in Brazil. I also believe that this discussion is in the end just one more attempt to answer the fundamental question of our time: How does one live with AIDS?

'AIDS' Before AIDS

The first impact of AIDS in Brazil was on the public imagination. Actually, it arrived as a 'feature section' virus, something which has not been without appreciable long-term consequences (Moraes and Carrara, 1985). Indeed, even today, I believe, the dominant ideas about AIDS stem from the ways in which the epidemic was first represented.

Even before any doctor had recorded a single verifiable case of AIDS, the press, especially the popular press, was presenting the arrival of the 'gay plague' in Brazil as inevitable. Expectations were generated and fanned, and there was even some fatalism. More than a few blew their alarmist trumpets to herald the arrival of punishment for sinners at last! Though there was discussion of how threatening AIDS could become in a country where public health provision was catastrophically deficient, and where infectious and parasitic diseases had never really been brought under control, no one doubted that AIDS would arrive. This epidemic, which was both real and remote, both deadly and sexual, both concrete and mysterious, was discussed primarily as a disease of 'others', not without an irony that frequently developed into the most merciless mockery.

The first banner headline on the 'gay plague' in Brazil surfaced in a newspaper called *Folha de O POVO*. This headline was not followed by a news story, but was printed as a joke for lack of any event with which to scandalize the paper's readers. The headline read: 'Gay Plague Leaves All the Faggots Closed-assed' (Daniel and Míccolis, 1983).[1] The problems with this headline were numerous. To begin with, the wording implied that there was panic among male homosexuals in Brazil, when in fact there was none. Few homosexuals in the large Brazilian cities at this time believed that the epidemic would affect them in any way. Second, the irreverence of the press, the unheeded concern of some health professionals, intellectuals and politicians, and also the indifference of the homosexual community reinforced the idea that AIDS was not a serious matter of concern to anyone.

If one reflects on this prehistory of AIDS in Brazil, it may be asked why the country did not prepare itself to check the epidemic when it first surfaced, since in many ways it was crystal clear that it would become very important. The new epidemic certainly created great agitation, but why did this not generate any action? I will argue that the adoption of an abstract and imported model, lacking relevance to the conditions of life in Brazil, proved an effective impetus to doing nothing at all.

Today, almost a decade later, when the cases are counted in the tens of thousands, it is disquieting to observe that now there is a kind of collective anaesthesia, made evident by the scant interest in AIDS from the new administration that took office in March 1990 — as if nothing more could be done in the face of an increasingly disastrous situation. To this day the government has taken no significant action in response to the epidemic, continuing the five-year record of inaction and indifference of the previous administration. There is today no adequate national program for controlling the epidemic, and the response of the previous administration, when there were already more than 1000 reported cases of AIDS, was a purely symbolic gesture. And so it remains. The idea that AIDS is inevitable (almost a price to be paid for the modernity of our cities), and the idea that it is not quite a Brazilian disease but something foreign or strange, has remained almost unchanged from the view that prevailed when AIDS arrived in Brazil. It is good not to forget what happened then, for we are experiencing the consequences of the attitudes that we took or failed to take at that time.

AIDS in Brazil: A False Model in Search of the 'Facts'

In societies in which modern means of communication predominate, rumour always moves faster than fact. Often, when a fact arrives, it is interpreted in the light of a rumour, which manages thereby to become more rather than less real. That is how it was with AIDS. More than once, the truth about this disease in Brazil had to be validated as true by the 'model' imported from the more industrialized countries of the north. An epidemic was announced that 'resembled' the American one. An epidemic was expected which would unfold according to the Western pattern. The preconceived model was looked for in doctors' offices and local epidemiological tables. Since it is not difficult to find the outcome of what a preconceived analysis is expected to produce, we ended up with a model that gave us an epidemiological pattern just like that of the first world. In Rio de Janeiro and New York, in São Paulo and San Francisco, it was the same AIDS. Above all, AIDS came to be regarded as a foreign disease in several senses. First, it was foreign in the lowest sense of all, xenophobia; it was a disease of American gays after all. Second, it was foreign in the sense that it did not fit the pattern of traditional epidemics (if there has ever been anywhere an epidemic that could be described as 'traditional'). Absurd as it might seem, these arguments were rehearsed even by government authorities, who asserted several times that AIDS was not a priority on the list of the country's common public health disasters.

To these authorities, AIDS at best was nothing more than an epidemic of 'minorities', simply a problem of a few rich and well-provided-for homosexuals. So long as AIDS was wreaking havoc only in these allegedly well defined 'risk groups', there was no reason to sound the alarm, no reason to alert that shapeless mass known as the 'general public'. It is important to note though that, according to the official arguments, what made AIDS less important was not that it was a disease of homosexuals but that it was a disease of 'rich' people. Several official declarations were released to the effect that according to official statistics the disease in Brazil attacked the upper crust, a 'fact' which flew in the face of the experience of all community groups and health professionals affected by the epidemic.

It was within this paradigm that AIDS was first investigated in Brazil. A 1988 study of the first 500 cases reported in Rio de Janeiro showed clearly how conformity to the North American model was generated by the structure of the survey's own questionnaire (see Guimarães *et al.*, 1988). One of the questions, for example, concerned 'risk trips' (which included trips abroad, chiefly to New York and San Francisco). That a case could be attributed to contagion from outside the country served as some degree of reassurance.

There was considerable difficulty, however, in fitting those first 500 cases into such 'risk groups' such as 'homosexuals' and 'bisexuals'. This terminology can scarcely be said to describe the common sexual practices between men in Brazil, which present more ambiguities than are dreamed of by an epidemiology borrowed from a society such as North America, where there actually is a gay community (see Chapter 4 in this volume). The richness of Brazilian sexual culture is not easily categorized along the lines of homosexuality, heterosexuality and bi-sexuality — classifications which establish a causal relationship between desire, the sexual act and sexual identity. In Brazil there are far more fluid criteria for establishing sexual identities. On the one hand, men that have sexual relations, occasionally or frequently, with other men continue to consider themselves 'men', both 'heterosexual' and 'macho', playing the active role in sexual relations. The social constructions that frame relations between the same sex can only be called 'homosexual' from a distance. On the other hand, there is nothing similar to a 'homosexual' or 'gay' community, in terms of the European and North American models (see Daniel and Míccolis, 1983; Fry, 1982; Fry and MacRae, 1983; Parker, 1989; Trevisan, 1986).

Given these realities, no wonder the questionnaire responses of the first 500 people with AIDS could not be easily codified. Usually the questionnaires were returned with the space for sexual practices studded with erasures. First a check mark would be entered in the space for 'heterosexual'; then that would be erased and another clearer check mark placed in the space for 'bisexual', and then a circle drawn around the word 'homosexual'. There were also arrows, marks and lines in different colours and intensities, attesting to the uncertainty of both interviewer and interviewee. There was no lack of dissatisfaction on the part of the interviewers, who, in addition to those three words, made a point of often entering a 'promiscuous' before the word 'homosexual'.

In addition, there was evidence of humour, some of it obscure to the interviewers. For example, one patient confessed to promiscuity, to having relations ten times a day, sometimes with cats, monkeys and parrots.[2] The interviewer was unacquainted with the common parlance of gay-identified men in Brazil, and thus missed the patient's joke (Fatal, 1988). The result was a fanciful instance of promiscuous bestiality that was no more than a colloquial leg-pull.

One feature of this inglorious study worthy of comment concerns the case of 'heterosexuals' suspected of infection through sexual contact, in which next to the word 'heterosexual' the term 'promiscuous' was written in red pencil. The advent of the 'promiscuous heterosexual', first identified in early 1987 (though not developed any further, since cases of 'promiscuous heterosexuals' are much rarer than others), demonstrates the logic of the preconceptions that operate within the dominant epidemiological model. While in time this mystery figure no longer commanded researchers' attention, the idea remained that promiscuity was one of the ways of acquiring AIDS.

Despite these difficulties, the model of AIDS in Brazil continued to be made to agree with that in the 'West'. One specific local characteristic was inserted, however. As it happened, at least one in five (20 per cent) of the AIDS cases recorded in those first five months of the epidemic had been caused by the use of contaminated blood or blood products. The issue of blood emerged then as a specific dimension within the epidemiological modelling of AIDS first in Rio de Janeiro and then elsewhere. This identified a more traditional public health catastrophe, caused by a contaminated blood supply, itself the result of an immoral trade controlling the blood market throughout the state. The magnitude of the numbers and the distribution of cases raised questions about the appropriateness of a purely 'Western' epidemiological model. Nevertheless, blood-related cases of infection came to be seen as a kind of exception, one that proved the rule concerning the overall relevance of the 'Western' model.

The tragedy that struck people with haemophilia and all other recipients of transfused blood in Rio de Janeiro in particular and in Brazil in general was insufficient to incite a reappraisal of existing epidemiological methods. It was sufficient, however, to alert the general public to AIDS and to generate a movement to protect the blood supply of the Brazilian people — strong enough even to secure the inclusion of important elements within the Constitution then being voted on. Today, for example, it is unconstitutional to trade in blood in Brazil. So far, however, this very well intentioned law remains unenforced by the public health authorities.

In summary, the adopted model anaesthetized awareness of the social problems revealed or exacerbated by AIDS. It continues to function as a camouflage: specific social and human problems can be blamed on an enigma and a mystery. As a result, 'knowledge' — such as that generated via medical and epidemiological research — becomes pure superstition, and the epidemic continues in its course, unfettered.

A 'Second-Class' Epidemic

In a perversion of policy, the false model ensured that AIDS was downgraded to a second-class epidemic, lacking the significance of the great epidemics of history that have never been eliminated. When it first appeared, and in the years that followed, AIDS was deemed such a small problem that even less provision was made against it.

Today two issues stand out when we consider the HIV/AIDS situation in Brazil. First is the growth of the epidemic to massive proportions. The growth of the number of cases is beginning to create difficulties in relation to the care of people with AIDS, especially because as AIDS starts to become more treatable, the question shifts from forced and painful survival — mere lingering in a hospital bed — to the complex issue of *living with AIDS*. Also growing, at a runaway pace, is the number of people with HIV infection who receive no care at all and lack even the basic information they need to deal with their own situation. Second, growing alongside the epidemic is the increasing impoverishment of people with AIDS. Brazil is a country where most of the population is needy and bereft of social services. It is inevitable, therefore, that AIDS should claim the largest number of people from this majority of the poor, mainly because they have no access to re-sources — whether material or symbolic: not only no hospitals, but also no education or information to help them cope with the disease.

In a few years we will probably be speaking of AIDS as a typical third world disease (including the third world pockets in more in-dustrialized countries). It will then have become just another 'traditional' epidemic. Just as it is now being treated by the authorities in Brazil, AIDS will be viewed as traditional by the world's medical community, a second-class epidemic, and by then the situation will be beyond re-demption, for, as it says in the Bible, mending cannot be done with old rags.

The World Is a Little Country

In Highland County, Virginia, there was much discussion about AIDS when E. Kuebler-Ross wanted to set up a home there for abandoned babies with AIDS. Much of the local community opposed the project, which could have hurt tourism, business and some other Christian sentiments and values. While the controversy raged, the local news-papers received numerous letters from readers (Kuebler-Ross, 1988). In one of them a woman who was probably very well informed wrote in block capitals, 'AIDS IS A WORLD PROBLEM'. Amid all the confused and prejudiced arguments of the local readers, this seemed a breath of the fresh air. But the woman went on to ask: 'SO WHY BRING IT TO HIGHLAND?'

Where is the world? Where does humanity start? AIDS, as a crisis of world society and the hallmark crisis of modern civilization, asks these questions in the most pragmatic of ways.

There can be no doubt that powerful ethnocentric sentiments prompt all societies to blame diseases on others. A familiar case is syphilis, which for Neapolitans was the French disease, and for the French the Neapolitan disease. Other examples abound. AIDS has added to the list of medically defined conditions ethnocentric and racist connotations. This is not the place to discuss the efforts to discover the origin of the virus. Whatever discoveries science may have made, the point is that there was always the certainty that the virus was alien, from outside, that is, from the third world, and before the third world, from the most alien world of all — wildlife, nature. Even when there were no proofs, this was the overriding conviction. The AIDS virus became stranger still after the dispute among scientists over who had discovered it (Leibowitch, 1984). It is well to note that while these historical discoveries can clear up some matters, they do not change the story of the epidemic as it is unfolding today. They in no way alter the fact that it began in large cities of the *Western* world as the epidemic we know today.

In any case, I mention this to underscore the general need to make a disease such as AIDS necessarily alien, something that entered society from 'outside', the result of a 'foreign' practice. One scientist study-ing the epidemic at the start was certain that American homosexuals had created, in saunas, bars and other unsanitary sex establishments, a 'sexual third world', as he called it, where diseases could multiply freely (Grmek, 1989). It must never have occurred to him that this sexual world was patently a product of the first world, of its large cities, of which the metropolises of the third world were merely poor imitations.

In reality, the AIDS epidemic is provoking a major economic breakdown, especially in third world countries. Brazil, for example, knows it does not have the means to surmount this crisis. In any case, no country can surmount the AIDS crisis if the epidemic is regarded as nothing more than a health crisis that can be dealt with by government and health system initiatives. Nor will we succeed if we cling to the official AIDS model in which pain — both physical and moral — becomes a central element of an economy that designates as 'society' only those who can produce, and removes from that core of citizenship those who cannot produce yet (children) and those who can produce no longer (the aged and the sick). In this view, production and the production of profit become the soul and essence of the citizen. Thus the city of men is the city of profit, of the quest for it and the worship of it. Human activity for production and reproduction outside this universe for the reproduction of consumer values is not a measurable economic quantity, and hence possesses no real human attributions. The irony is that if we fail to consider these 'unmeasurables', the social and economic devastation brought about by AIDS will be beyond reckoning.

If the epidemic is seen as a vast crisis of society, then it is obvious that measures against AIDS must be constructed around a clear idea of citizenship and hence of solidarity. To deal with this disease, we must rally major resources in the community. If AIDS is viewed only as a private, 'individual matter', or even only as the attribute of 'groups', the most that will happen is an effort to provide care in order to minimize the effects of the problem. There will be no mobilization of the community so long as the disease is not seen as a global problem, a collective obligation.

From a cold analytical standpoint it might appear that ideas of solidarity are effective merely in a humanitarian sense, an attitude that is more poetic than practical. More than poetic, however, and for good reason, solidarity is primarily a political attitude, a conception of democracy as a day-to-day condition, a precondition for and a definition of citizenship.

Here the effectiveness — or rather the ineffectiveness — of the abstract model adopted for AIDS exposes its economic consequences. First, it does not allow us to control the epidemic and facilitates a course that will make it impossible to do anything later except to tally up the losses. Second, it encourages us to view the person with AIDS as legally dead, and all that is left to do is to wait for him or her physically to die. The relegated sufferer is not enlisted in an effort of primary importance, which is to prevent the epidemic. Surely the mobilization of people who live with HIV is vital (in more than one sense) for lessening the impact of the epidemic on a community? Finally, the model discriminates instead of encouraging participation. For these reasons alone, solidarity is a necessary response in this epoch of AIDS.

AIDS and Aids: Lives Before and With

Who is living with AIDS? At least those diagnosed as having the opportunistic diseases that result from the immunodeficiency caused by the human immunodeficiency viruses. But since the advent of the relevant tests, we have known about the seropositive individual who carries the antibodies to the viruses in her or his body and lives with few or minimal symptoms of the longer-term infection. Those who may be classed in the general category of virus carriers are many, in the millions (worldwide, the World Health Organization estimated between 6 and 10 million at the beginning of the 1990s [World Health Organization, 1990]). Many more are linked to those who are HIV antibody positive by the most diverse human bonds: they are parents, children, brothers, relatives, lovers, spouses and sweethearts, friends and acquaintances, neighbours or — simply and yet more complexly — contemporaries. These are the many millions more that the virus has encountered in its path. Who can say that these people, directly involved as they are, are not living with AIDS? Here I am certainly not talking about medical definitions, but about a complex social structure that requires a new term to try to encompass the vast field of intended meaning. I am talking about 'aids', a common noun that refers to a complex of epidemics with a far wider social impact than a mere diagnosis that may be made through tests on an individual body or even on millions of such bodies.

To determine who is living with aids today is a problem that cannot be solved in the laboratory. No blood test can determine who is living with aids. While such a test can detect antibodies or viruses in the bloodstream, it cannot show the established antibody of solidarity and its varieties — and of its contraries — in everyday life today. HIV is following its biological course while another complex of virulences (we could simply call them ideological viruses) has spread through the social structure of aids, developing it into a three-dimensional photograph of contemporary civilization. Thus it is no metaphor to assert that, on the planetary scale, humankind is seropositive. It is a historical and political axiom that merits extensive explanation.

In its medical, epidemiological and sociological sense, AIDS (used in the broad sense, as covering the whole infectious process caused by HIV) has set off a health crisis without precedent and has thus become the direst challenge to science at the end of the century. Aids, however (understood here as the whole breadth of the social structure that I label with the term in lower case letters), is not a problem of science or health. It is a crisis of society. The terms of the equation that can express it are political and ideological unknowns, and at its root is the complex idea of solidarity.

The AIDS model overlaps with highly distinctive features of modern life: the economic and political unification of the planet, and the sharpness of its economic and political divisions; the physical world is progressively smaller and its social distances ever greater; the change in the power of medicine, in which we are already witnessing the demise of the clinic; the innovation of technologies of power; the emergence of new rights.

I Have AIDS. I'm Alive

They say that telling one's story can save lives. Perhaps because it creates an awareness of risk, perhaps because it mobilizes solidarity, and perhaps simply because it breathes life into some benumbed feeling. I have many doubts about such claims. I am not sure that telling one's story is all that effective and redeeming. In my lifetime I have seen that experience itself never educates nor enhances until it has passed through the screen of the critical consciousness. I do not, therefore, aspire to that purpose, I have decided to write about living with AIDS in order to say just one thing: I'm alive. No, this is not going to help save lives — not even mine. No, telling the story is *not* going to help save lives. But it may improve some, or improve life in general. That is why people write, or else it would make no sense just to add one's own mundane observations to the general fund of triviality.

I know that many are telling immensely detailed stories about all the contests that are being waged inside their bodies. Some approach life with the virus as a kind of battle, and know they are going to 'lose' the war. I cannot see myself as contending with a biological virus. I do not think I am ever going to lose any war in this way. I am certain, first of all, that aids would defeat me if I entered into the metaphor of war. AIDS — here I mean the opportunistic diseases that the immunodeficiency caused by HIV allows to intervene — can kill. Certainly it causes many hardships, and can even go so far as to immobilize me totally or partially for a long time — either temporarily or permanently. It would defeat me not by killing me, but if I abandoned the awareness that I *live* with it and must adapt to certain circumstances of life imposed by it.

I do not claim to have a solution for those who have to deal with aids, but I am certain that the solution can only be found if those who live with it start to take a hand in solving the problem of the epidemic. As individuals, we are very unlikely to find much to alleviate our burden, though matters become easier if we are more aware of aids in its broader dimensions. For those who see AIDS only as a war, the only armistice they can envisage is a cure, which first requires a peace treaty signed by others as well as oneself. The war unfolds in the form of an effort by physicians contending with the virus and the operation of other more or less sophisticated technologies in the available arsenal.

I am not a battlefield. I am not a landscape, but rather the presence that is significant in the landscape my body has become in this illness. There is no chance of victories or defeats on this field. There are other possibilities, however — of wisdom or stupidity, love or hate, greatness or meanness, solidarity or persecution.

In these days of my life I have discovered that life is the discovery of fragility. I am living day by day and I am able to live — with an avidity not at all uncertain, but certainly undirected, like a hunger that should have started a millennium ago if I had only known then the millennial pleasures of each second that the intensity of life provides.

The World of Life — Almost the End

The argument put forward by the woman of Highland County reminded me of a Woody Allen film in which a child suffering from anxiety is taken by his mother to a psychiatrist because of his strange ideas. The child is bewildered because he has discovered that the universe is expanding. His mother scolds him and tells him that he has nothing to worry about because Brooklyn is *not* expanding.

I do not live in Highland. I have always lived in countries — if I ever 'lived' in any country — where the world's problems happen on my doorstep, at the end of my street, within a radius of 100 metres from my navel, close to where I live. I have always lived in places where the world's problems intruded upon me not just through the screen of the television set or the pages of the newspapers. These problems have taken immediate form in real people and the inevitable movements of things and beings around me. They have become concrete accretions of the whole planet within my own body cells.

I am a citizen of the third world, but I am certain that Highland is not far away. Highland is today, and everywhere. It is a little town deep in the state of Rio de Janeiro where a young woman who had been the domestic servant of a homosexual man was 'accused' of having AIDS and then of spreading the virus by mixing her blood in the children's ketchup in supermarkets. It is a little town in the northeast of Brazil where a homosexual man was driven out under several charges, including that of having been seen 'touching several fruits at the open-air market' with the obvious intention, as his accusers charged, of spreading infection. Highland is the downtown area of the cosmopolitan city of São Paulo, where the Grupo Pela VIDDA (Group for LIFE — for the Value, Integration and Dignity of the Person with AIDS), of which I am a member, encountered enormous difficulty renting a room for its headquarters, because its members have AIDS. Highland is the kind of environment in which the AIDS epidemic is at its worst, where the epidemic is a coldly economic matter of health. Highland, which that woman wanted to keep uninvolved with the world aids problem, is one of the innumerable capitals of the epidemic in the world. Highland is within all of us. This is the dominant response to our distress and our defeat by the epidemic of emotional plagues which AIDS has brought with it.

I am taking inventory here of a collective pain. The pain becomes laceration when fertilized in the garden of indifference, in the landscape of intolerance. Highland, in the end, is Brazil as well, where the 'poor' die more often than the rich, and will die of AIDS much faster than the rich. Where we have no sure count of the number of AIDS cases because the figures are not just muddled, but falsified as well (ABIA, 1989). Where we do not know what AIDS is doing because there are no surveys. Where people with AIDS die at the doorsteps of hospitals that were neglected during the years of the authoritarian military regime and are today powerless to cope with the catastrophic breakdown of public health throughout the country. Where the people do not believe in AIDS because the information they receive refers to a metaphorical disease that is full of mysteries. Where even today it has yet to be *proven*, even to gay men, that there is such a thing as an AIDS epidemic, and not just a CIA plot to wipe out all gays, or a device of the newspapers to encourage their persecution. Where there is a need to educate physicians who know nothing about the disease, and teachers, prelates and authorities, to make them see that AIDS is not a punishment from heaven. Where $200,000 worth of HIV antibody test materials had to be thrown away because they had passed their expiration, where another unspecified quantity of AZT, also expired, is discarded because it was bought by the Ministry of Health but lost in the corridors of the blasted bureaucracy. Where people die of opportunistic infections for which there are no available cures because of bureaucratic problems affecting the import of experimental treatment drugs. Where no legal aid of any kind is provided for people with HIV, and the legal department of an organization such as the Grupo Pela VIDDA has to handle the legal affairs of hundreds of persons in order to defend basic legal rights acquired by the population decades ago, at least on paper, and especially in matters of employment. Where citizenship is regarded as a luxury, and people with HIV/AIDS are condemned to a silent form of legal death with the kind complicity of the government authorities. Where health authorities say in the press that AZT should not be purchased for patients in public hospitals because 'they're going to die anyway.'

But Brazil is also a country where thousands of people rally heroically in community organizations without funds or support so there will be more than just despair. I am writing a testament not only of pain, but also of compassion. In speaking of those who are holding on, of the revolt of dignity, I must say that every string of calamities consolidates yet further a strategy of solidarity. The world is everywhere. And the better world is the one we will build in our hearts by making our arms into aerial roots, and linking ourselves each to the other.

A response to aids on behalf of *life* entails national and local programming ranging from funding to meet the material needs of a growing population, to the mobilization of social and human resources to guarantee the full exercise of people's rights as citizens. Aids cannot be spoken of as a problem *on* the planet. The epidemic is a fact *of* the planet. This fact is part of the struggle for the 'defence of life'. The fight against aids is of the same order of importance as the defence of life on the planet. The issue of human rights, viewed in its larger dimension as a broad democratic matter calling for the practice of solidarity, is the greatest challenge of the 1990s, mainly in countries such as Brazil, where representative democracy is still in its infancy.

We are living and learning with AIDS and with aids. We can infect every country on the planet with the most extreme and inexorable epidemic known to humanity: *life*. Let us hope that this will be our greatest impact, so that in the coming century we may be remembered as more than just contemporaries of infamy — as the precursors of a world in which the human condition is not just the triumph of the absurd. There are still millions of stars alive within the cosmos. LONG LIVE LIFE!

Notes

1 This headline is written in a vulgar and extremely insulting language. It is quoted in the text specifically for its grotesque humour and for the profound disrespect that is contained therein.
2 The expression 'cats, monkeys and parrots' comes from a popular way to identify the family, with all its institutions, through an ironic and allegorical enumeration of all the members, close and distant relatives, and even the prized animals. So this enumeration of the most common domestic animals means, metaphorically, a certain excess, or 'a bit of everything'. It is almost a way of saying 'etc.' in a humorous way.

Chapter 3

The Third Epidemic:
An Exercise in Solidarity

Herbert Daniel and Richard Parker

In the late 1980s Jonathan Mann, who was at the time the Director of the World Health Organization's Global Programme on AIDS, suggested that it is possible to distinguish between at least three phases of the AIDS epidemic in any given community — three phases that are so distinct that they can be described as three different epidemics. The first is the epidemic of HIV infection that silently enters the community and often proceeds almost unnoticed. The second epidemic, after a delay of a number of years, is the epidemic of AIDS itself: the syndrome of infectious diseases that can occur because of HIV infection. Finally, the third (perhaps most potentially explosive) epidemic is the epidemic of social, cultural, economic and political reactions to AIDS — reactions that, in Mann's words, are 'as central to the global AIDS challenge as the disease itself' (see Mann, 1987; Panos Institute, 1988, 1990; Sabatier, 1988).

This chapter focuses on the third AIDS epidemic in Brazil. It examines some of the complicated, and sometimes contradictory, reactions and responses that have emerged since 1982, when the first cases of AIDS were reported in Brazil and the disease itself began to enter Brazilian consciousness as one of the most serious health problems in contemporary life. This third epidemic, in Brazil as elsewhere, is clearly linked to the epidemics of HIV infection and AIDS. Yet the relationship is often a complex one, as the reactions of Brazilian society in the face of these first two epidemics have often been based on largely distorted images of what AIDS is, whom it affects, and how it affects them.

Together with these specific images, the wider social reaction to AIDS in Brazil has been shaped within a context in which even the most basic health problems faced by the population as a whole have never been fully confronted or resolved (ABIA, 1988b). Brazil is a country in which endemic diseases of traditional rural life, accentuated by economic underdevelopment, continue to exist alongside the more modern diseases of a rapidly industrializing society — a country in which the notion of public health has long been viewed as an almost insoluble problem. On top of this, during twenty years of authoritarian military government between 1964 and 1984, the privatization of the medical system created a clear deterioration of the basic medical services available to the general public. To speak of a 'calamitous health picture' in Brazil has became commonplace, and has often masked a defeatist attitude suggesting that little or nothing can be done in the face of such overwhelming health problems.

Within this setting the AIDS epidemic has often been presented, even by successive Ministers of Health and other high ranking health officials, as a secondary problem — relatively insignificant in comparison with more complex, statistically significant dilemmas. The potential seriousness of the epidemic has been minimized further still by a vision that focuses on the person with AIDS as part of a social minority — on the one hand, as a member of some limited 'elite', yet on the other hand, as fundamentally 'marginal' within the wider structure of society. These distorted analyses, in turn, have largely shaped the official policies aimed at controlling the AIDS epidemic.

The result of such distortions, in Brazil as in so many other societies, has all too often been one of prejudice, discrimination and sometimes even violence. Based on partial understandings and outright misunderstandings, the reactions not only of individuals, but even of social groups and institutions, in the face of AIDS, have frequently been motivated by fear more than anything else. They have resulted less in reasonable and responsible collective action aimed at confronting the epidemic than in what might be described as a syndrome of blame and accusation that has ultimately done little to slow the spread of HIV infection or to provide care for those affected by AIDS.

Even if this has been the dominant reaction in the face of AIDS, however, some hope can nonetheless be found in the fact that it has not gone unquestioned. In Brazil, as in so many other parts of the world in recent years, this fundamentally reactionary response has increasingly been contested, and the task of fashioning a more informed, positive response in the future has become the central goal of a growing number of voluntary groups and professional organizations. In the face of prejudice and fear, information and social solidarity have increasingly been identified as the only truly effective response to the spread of AIDS.

This chapter is itself a product of, and a contribution to, this more recent counter-response in the face of AIDS. Our goal is to analyze critically some of the significant forces that have shaped the third epidemic, and by doing so, to contribute to the development of a more informed future response. With this in mind, we have divided the body of the text into three major sections. First, we analyze what might be described as some of the major myths or fallacies that have been constructed around and about the AIDS epidemic — images of the disease and its so-called 'victims' that have shaped an initial climate of fear and prejudice. Second, we move from this climate to some of the concrete acts and incidences of violence and discrimination that have marked the social history of AIDS in Brazil. Third, we examine some of the recent developments in the Brazilian fight against AIDS — in particular, the emergence of groups and organizations aimed at responding more effectively to the epidemic. Finally, in a brief concluding section, we bring these various discussions together to give some sense of where we believe this third AIDS epidemic is going — how it is spreading, and what its future will be in Brazil.

Images of AIDS

While we now know that the silent spread of HIV in the Brazilian population was taking place at least as early as the late 1970s, it was only in 1982, with the first reported cases of AIDS in Brazil, that the third epidemic gradually began to take shape in contemporary Brazilian life. Even before AIDS had become statistically significant, however, it had attracted widespread attention, particularly in the mass media, and, by extension, had become a major topic for conversation even in daily life. Long before most Brazilians had any direct contact with the disease, then, they had already formed complex, and often contradictory, understandings of it — understandings based largely on the images and representations of AIDS and its perceived 'victims' that had been produced and reproduced in the media and then extended and developed in the discourses of daily life.

Over the course of a number of years at least two interrelated sets of images have been particularly important in shaping the wider social response to AIDS in Brazil. On the one hand, central attention has focused on the 'victims' of AIDS, and an understanding of the epidemic as a whole has been predicated on a whole range of assumptions concerning the perceived nature of those who are directly affected by it. On the other hand, on top of this focus on its victims yet another

set of assumptions has been built up concerning the most basic characteristics of the disease itself. Mixing popular prejudices and scientific
theories in ways that have often made it impossible to distinguish one
from the other, these different representations seem to have played
into one another across time, reinforcing one another and profoundly
influencing the ways in which Brazilian society has responded to the
epidemic.

During the earliest years of the epidemic it was perhaps above all
else the perceived nature of its 'victims' that dominated public attention. In Brazil, as in the United States and Western Europe, the vast
majority of the earliest AIDS cases were reported among homosexual
men, many of whom had spent extensive time living or travelling
outside Brazil, and who were thus thought to have been infected with
HIV while abroad. As an extension of this, they were generally thought
to be relatively well-to-do individuals who divided their time between
Rio de Janeiro or São Paulo and foreign centres such as New York
or Paris. Perhaps even more important, they were almost uniformly
characterized in terms of their 'promiscuous' sexual conduct — a kind
of dangerous immorality that quickly became central to the popular
understanding of AIDS (see Daniel, 1985; Galvão, 1985; Morães and
Carrara, 1985).

Although the extent to which this image of people with AIDS
offered an accurate picture of some kind of underlying epidemiological
reality was rarely raised, even by medical experts and public health
officials, it nonetheless dominated early discussion of the epidemic,
and has continued to play a central role in the popular understanding
of AIDS. As in parts of Europe and the United States, the epidemic
quickly took shape (in what might be described as the social imagination)
as a kind of *'praga gay'* or 'gay plague' that was basically limited to
what was already one of the most clearly marginalized segments of
contemporary Brazilian society. Linked, as it was, in turn, with the
lives of a relatively few, well travelled and well-to-do individuals, it
could quite easily be written off, even by the highest ranking public
health officials, as a disease of but a limited elite that required little in
the way of government action and no significant commitment of
financial resources (*Folha de São Paulo*, 1988a).

Even by the mid-1980s the gradually emerging understanding of
the epidemiology of AIDS in Brazil had made this view of the epidemic
altogether untenable. On the contrary, while homosexual contacts continued to account for the highest number of reported AIDS cases,
they nonetheless constituted less than half of the cases reported as a
whole; and the number of cases linked to both bisexual and heterosexual

contacts, on the one hand, and to contact with contaminated blood and blood products, on the other hand, had quickly emerged as equally significant factors in the spread of the Brazilian AIDS epidemic. In addition, research aimed at investigating the social background of people with AIDS and the sociological profile of the epidemic had demonstrated the degree to which the spread of HIV infection in fact cut across class and status boundaries, taking perhaps its greatest toll on the poorest segments of Brazilian society (ABIA, 1988a).

Even in the face of significant contrary evidence, however, the view of AIDS as homosexual disease, and all of the stigmas related to homosexuality itself, has continued to have a major impact in shaping the Brazilian response to the epidemic. Even as the exclusively homosexual focus has been called into question, this initial view, with its central emphasis on the fundamental marginality of those affected by HIV/AIDS, seems to have served as a model for the gradual expansion of the epidemic within the popular imagination. Images of middle- or upper-class homosexuals have given way to a whole new cast of characters — characters who are linked to this earlier view above all else by their social and moral marginality. Prostitutes, prisoners, transvestites, street children and drug addicts, for example, have all taken their place alongside homosexuals within the imagery conjured up by the mention of AIDS, and have become part of an ever-expanding vision not only of marginality, but, by extension, of danger. Still characterized as a disease of the elite, AIDS has simultaneously begun to take shape as an affliction of the underclass — of the poorest and, ultimately, most dangerously threatening segments of Brazilian society.

This basic characterization of the 'AIDS victim', and, by extension, of those most at risk in the face of the epidemic, has ultimately been linked to a wider pattern of meanings in which social marginality is quickly translated into a whole series of notions related to contamination, contagion and danger. Particularly in highly hierarchical social settings such as contemporary Brazil, the most marginalized sectors of society have long been seen as a source of danger, and have traditionally been subject to a whole range of practices aimed at both moral and physical containment and control. It is perhaps hardly surprising, then, in the light of these connections, that people with AIDS, and even those thought to be potentially at risk of HIV infection, have often become the focus for irrational fear and prejudice.

Unfortunately, this situation has only been accentuated by yet another set of images related not so much to people with AIDS as to the disease itself. Since the epidemic first began to take shape, particularly on the pages of daily newspapers, the perceived marginality of its so-called victims has been linked to the perceived severity of its apparent consequences. Central attention has focused, perhaps above all else, on at least three characteristics of the disease: its contagious nature, its apparent incurability, and its inevitably fatal outcome. Taken together, these (obviously interrelated) characteristics have come to constitute an essentially minimal definition of what AIDS is — a definition that may well represent certain scientific facts, but that has ultimately led to the abuse of basic human rights (Daniel, 1989).

Perhaps more than anything else, it is the contagious nature of the disease that has captured popular attention — the fact that AIDS 'spreads', that it can be caught, and that one gets it through one's contacts with others. Linking complex notions of sickness, filth or contamination, and sexual perversion, AIDS has tied this notion of contagion to the dangerous transgression implied in prohibited practices such as sex or drug use. Like the moral contagion of its marginal victims, AIDS somehow rubs off — it contaminates even the most apparently 'innocent' victims who unwittingly come into contact with it. The fact that HIV is transmitted only through a relatively limited, and relatively well known, number of ways, however, has all too often been forgotten, as attention has focused almost hysterically at times on the principle of 'contagion' (rather than a rational analysis of the concrete modes of transmission) as central to the image of HIV and AIDS.

Much the same somewhat distorted emphasis has been linked, as well, to the ultimate effects of the disease. Unlike less severe ailments, it has been repeatedly stressed, AIDS offers those affected no hope of cure, and its incurability has become central to virtually all of the most basic popular understandings of the disease as a whole. AIDS is understood as an inevitably fatal disease in which even an initial diagnosis translates directly into a sentence of death — a disease in which the very social being of those it affects is therefore called into question, their citizenship placed within parentheses (see Sontag, 1977, 1989). Again, rather less attention has focused on what might be described as the quality of life of people with AIDS, as the ultimate consequence of an untimely death has dominated the discussion of the epidemic.

Ultimately, then, AIDS has taken shape as very much a special case — a disease unlike other diseases whose perceived victims are unlike other victims. Like leprosy, it quite literally defines the very being of those affected: not simply *'pessoas com AIDS'* ('people with AIDS') in Brazil, but *'Aidéticos'* ('Aidetics'). Built up, in popular conception, as larger than life and synonymous with death, AIDS has taken shape in Brazil, as elsewhere, as part of a context in which the most basic principles of human rights can somehow cease to exist or hold true. Distorted images of both AIDS and those affected by it have dominated the public discussion of the epidemic, and have all too often produced the kind of moral panic (see Weeks, 1985; Watney,1987) that almost inevitably ignores or violates the rights and humanity of a stigmatized minority. It is against this background, unfortunately, that the social history of AIDS in Brazil has most clearly been played out, and it is to some of its most obvious (even if unintended) consequences that we now turn.

The Consequences of Fear and Prejudice

Precisely because the AIDS epidemic took shape in the mass media and in popular conception even before it had actually affected the lives of significant numbers of individuals, and because the popular under- standing of the epidemic has so often been based on misinformation and distortion, it is perhaps hardly surprising that from the very start the most basic social response to AIDS should have been one of panic and fear. The earliest widely reported cases of AIDS seem to have almost inevitably given rise to acts of oppression or inhumanity. In the interior of Minas Gerais a young man who had returned home after contracting HIV in Rio de Janeiro was stoned out of town. In large cities such as Rio or São Paulo people with AIDS were frequently refused admission to local hospitals, and were sometimes left lying at the emergency entrance for hours while their relatives tried to arrange for permission to have them attended to. Ambulance drivers refused to transport suspected people with HIV/AIDS, and even highly trained medical personnel were sometimes responsible for disseminating in- accurate and misleading information about the nature of AIDS and its prospective impact in Brazilian society (see Trevisan, 1986; *Veja*, 1985a, 1985b).

Specific incidents of cruelty and inhumanity are unfortunately all too easy to list. What is perhaps most important, however, is to under- stand the ways in which such incidents become linked together as part of a broader social and cultural configuration — a configuration in which the distorted images, of both the disease and those it affects, that we have already discussed seem to have become linked to pre-existing prejudices in ways that ultimately reproduce and reinvent these prejudices as the only available response to the epidemic. AIDS has thus emerged, for example, as a readily available legitimation for the oppression of already stigmatized groups such as prostitutes or homosexual men, and police raids directed against well known gay meeting places, or, in one widely publicized case, areas that serve as a focus for transvestite prostitution, have been presented by the authorities as efforts aimed at AIDS prevention. Police violence here pretends to serve the interests of the public health (*Folha de São Paulo*, 1987).

This kind of basic confusion between images of male homosexuality and images of AIDS has perhaps been especially problematic within the medical profession, where long-standing misunderstandings in relation to homosexual lifestyles have quickly translated into a new set of misunderstandings related to AIDS (see Mott, 1987). On the one hand, individuals classified as homosexuals have automatically been linked to AIDS regardless of related circumstances, as in one case in which the patient's homosexuality, linked to what appeared to be an AIDS-related infection, was enough to elicit an AIDS diagnosis without any associated testing to confirm the diagnosis (let alone counselling concerning its implications). In almost the reverse case, another patient, suffering from two severe AIDS-related disorders, was never tested for antibodies to HIV simply because his homosexual behaviour was unknown to his doctor and family members, and the possibility that he might be suffering from what is still perceived as a homosexual disease never entered their minds. In short, faced with a lack of understanding about both homosexuality and AIDS, not only the general public, but even the medical profession have ultimately relied on preconceived notions and outright fantasies that often have little to do with reality but that result in altogether inadequate treatment and care.

Just as pre-existing notions and prejudices relating to male homosexuality have shaped the treatment of AIDS, the stigmatization of other groups perceived to be at risk due to HIV infection has frequently led to various forms of discrimination. Doctors who work with street people, prostitutes and transvestites in Rio de Janeiro, for example, report hostile reactions on the part of their medical colleagues as they themselves, apparently through guilt by association, come to be seen as sources of contagion and risk. When they send their patients to clinics at local hospitals, the patient's simple appearance is enough to require that he or she must confront the aggressive questioning of a whole string of secretaries, social workers and nurses before gaining entry even for a simple examination. Since the emergence of AIDS, and its widely publicized association with transvestite prostitution, it has become virtually impossible to find medical personnel willing to participate even in relatively basic surgical procedures (such as appendectomy) on transvestite patients. Not surprisingly, in the face of such extensive discrimination, more than a few individuals give up in despair without receiving the medical attention that they require. Among such stigmatized groups the number of PWAs who have died alone, in their homes and without any medical assistance, is tragically climbing.

Like preconceived images of stigmatized or marginalized practices such as homosexuality, prostitution or transvestism, the whole notion of contagion in relation to AIDS seems to have given rise, as well, to almost hysterical responses in a wide range of different settings. In a society that still suffers from infectious diseases such as malaria, for example, the scientifically invalid assumption that HIV might be transmitted by mosquitos continues to exercise a powerful hold on the popular imagination. In at least one instance, in a small city in northeastern Brazil, it provided the focus for an organized campaign on the part of the local citizens aimed at preventing the return of a resident with AIDS whose presence, it was thought, might open the way for a local epidemic borne by mosquitos. No less problematic, throughout the course of the epidemic, significant public attention has focused on individuals (especially those who are marginal or marginalized) who are thought wilfully to seek to contaminate others, for example, by knowingly sharing contaminated needles or by seeking to engage in sexual contacts aimed at spreading HIV (*Washington Post*, 1987; *Jornal do Brasil*, 1988).

While these examples may seem extreme, what is particularly important about them, and about the widespread attention that they have received throughout Brazilian society, is the extent to which they create a moral climate conducive not merely to exaggerated paranoia, but to a generalized (and sometimes all too specific) discrimination against people with AIDS — as well as against those individuals who are perceived to be at risk of HIV. This, in turn, has created a situation in which precisely those people who are potentially at risk are perhaps those who are least likely (or able) to seek the information and assistance that they require. With relatively little in the way an organized gay community able to provide information and support in a positive setting, individuals involved in same-sex practices must generally rely upon the same medical and governmental institutions that have traditionally stigmatized and oppressed them, and have little reason to trust in or cooperate with these authorities. Even though the single most significant rise in the transmission of HIV in recent years has been among injecting drug users, clinics for the treatment of drug use refuse to accept AIDS patients and have even begun to require negative HIV antibody tests as a criterion for admission, making it practically impossible for those who need it most to receive treatment (*Veja*, 1989).

As this dilemma might suggest, in Brazil as in a number of other countries, blood testing has itself become a major point of contention, and has perhaps accentuated the growing chasm that seems to have been created between the authorities charged with confronting the AIDS epidemic and the men and women most at risk of HIV. While voluntary HIV blood testing might potentially serve as a useful tool in combatting the epidemic, virtually no free, anonymous testing sites are available or equipped with adequate psychological counselling services. Individuals involved in practices or behaviours that place them at risk must thus choose between living with the uncertainty of remaining untested and what they may well perceive to be the even greater risk of being tested under circumstances that may protect neither their confidentiality nor their basic human rights. At the same time that resources for adequate voluntary blood testing are lacking, however, the mandatory screening of populations such as prisoners or interned and abandoned children goes ahead in many institutions, even if with little evidence of a positive or productive payback (*Folha de São Paulo*, 1988b). A complex set of political questions has thus begun to take shape over the most effective manner to confront the epidemic, particularly in relation to troublesome issues such as blood testing, but the most basic response, thus far at least, seems to have generated conflict and distrust rather than cooperation and solidarity.

From the very beginning, then, the history of AIDS in Brazil, as in so many other nations, has been marked by fear, prejudice and injustice — a syndrome of blame and accusation that is ultimately every bit as dangerous as the more widely publicized syndrome of acquired immunodeficiency (Daniel, 1985). Yet even here things are not perhaps as simple as they seem, and the evolving situation has grown increasing complex and varied. Indeed, in virtually every case that we have noted, from attacks on transvestite prostitutes to unfounded concerns about mosquitos, irrational and inhumane responses on the part of some have quickly generated counter-responses on the part of others. Increasingly over the course of recent years, AIDS has become a point of contention within society, and misinformation has been confronted with information as Brazilian society has gradually sought to work through the incredibly difficult issues that AIDS has raised. In a sense AIDS itself has become a focus not only for the oppressive exercise of power, but also for resistance, and slowly but also surely, what we might describe as a politics of AIDS has gradually begun to emerge. While the struggle for a more adequate response to the AIDS epidemic in Brazil is only just beginning, the fact that it is beginning, and that it is being carried out on a number of fronts, offers perhaps the greatest hope for the future.

Toward a Politics of AIDS in Brazil

Understanding the emergence of AIDS as a political issue in Brazil is possible only if we remember that the development of the AIDS epidemic has taken place within a wider historical context — that it has occurred at precisely the same time that Brazilian society has sought to take the first tentative steps toward the re-establishment of a participatory democracy after two full decades of authoritarian rule (see ABIA, 1988b; Parker, 1993; see also Chapter 1 in this volume).

The impact of this wider context cannot be stated strongly enough, as it structured an initial situation in which the very tradition of citizenship (which has always been at least somewhat contested in Brazilian history), and the active involvement of the citizenry in the events and decisions of the wider society, had been systematically repressed — repressed, in many cases, during the entire lifetime of a major segment of the population in what is an overwhelmingly young nation. If the syndrome of blame and accusation characterizing the early response to AIDS in Brazil has tended to place within parentheses, as we have suggested, the very citizenship of people with AIDS or at risk because of AIDS, it is perhaps hardly surprising that this should have received relatively little attention — for twenty years Brazilians had lived under a political regime in which the citizenship of virtually the entire population had been placed within parentheses. Indeed, more surprising is the fact that gradually, in recent years, this syndrome of prejudice, and the violation of fundamental human rights and human dignity that it has so often produced, has been called into question by individuals and groups that have begun to form in order to fight against it (ABIA, 1988b).

On the one hand, significant work has begun to be carried out by already existing groups such as the Associação dos Hemofílicos (Haemophilia Association) and gay organizations such as Atobá or GGB (the Gay Group of Bahia), who have responded to the perceived risk among their different clienteles by becoming involved in political organizing around AIDS-related issues as well as in disseminating educational materials. On the other hand, any number of new groups or organizations have been formed specifically in response to AIDS since mid-1985, when a diverse group of people, ranging from health practitioners to community activists and members of gay organizations, came together in São Paulo to form GAPA (the Support Group for the Prevention of AIDS), a voluntary organization aimed at providing primary care and counselling services to people with AIDS as well as educating and informing the general public.

Since its initial organization in São Paulo, the membership and activities of GAPA have grown steadily, and essentially independent chapters have been founded in Rio de Janeiro, Belo Horizonte and half a dozen other major centres. In addition, shortly after the foundation of GAPA, leading intellectuals came together in Rio to form ABIA (the Brazilian Interdisciplinary AIDS Association), aimed at gathering and channelling information on AIDS throughout the country, at producing educational and informational materials, and at engaging in a constructive critique of government policy as a central part of elaborating more informed public health initiatives. Indeed, over the course of two years a whole range of other organizations have followed; and the work of groups such as GAPA and ABIA has been carried on in a variety of other directions by groups such as ARCA (Religious Support against AIDS), an ecumenical group of religious leaders, or the Grupo Pela VIDDA (the Group for LIFE), formed principally by people with HIV or AIDS, their friends and relatives, who are working to defend the human and civil rights of people with AIDS in Brazilian society.

During the past five years these diverse groups and organizations have gradually begun to open up important new ground in the struggle against AIDS in Brazil — to create what might be described as a politics of AIDS aimed at confronting not only the epidemics of HIV infection and AIDS, but also the third epidemic of prejudice and blame. They have been at the forefront in denouncing discrimination against both people with AIDS and people perceived to be at risk due to AIDS, and have focused, perhaps above all else, on combatting the effects of stigmatization and marginalization. Ultimately, they have offered, in contrast, the notion of '*solidariedade*' or 'solidarity' as the only truly acceptable response to AIDS — as central to the struggle against AIDS not only in Brazil but internationally as well — and have thus taken perhaps the first tentative steps toward rewriting the history of AIDS in contemporary Brazilian life.

Conclusion

At this point we can offer only a preliminary interpretation of the third epidemic as it has taken shape in Brazil — some sense of where the epidemic has been, but only a partial view of where it might go. The initial response of Brazilian society in the face of the epidemics of HIV and AIDS has been at best mixed. Distorted understandings, and outright misunderstandings, concerning the nature and impact of both HIV and AIDS have all too often led to a climate of fear and blame, to specific acts of cruelty and discrimination. Yet the fact that fear and injustice have themselves given rise to an increasingly vocal and organized opposition aimed at shaping a more just and humane response to AIDS, and to the people whose lives it most obviously touches, offers a significant degree of hope that it may be possible to shape a better future.

This goal is centrally important not only because it is the only ethically and morally acceptable one, but also because, even in the most explicitly pragmatic terms, it is ultimately the only viable response to the AIDS epidemic. As Jonathan Mann pointed out in suggesting the very distinction among three epidemics, or three phases of the broader AIDS epidemic, the argument that discrimination against individuals infected with or at risk in the face of HIV is somehow justified by the need to protect the broader public health is a fallacious one. On the contrary, the protection of the uninfected is fundamentally dependent upon the preservation of the rights and dignity of those already infected. The battle against AIDS depends upon overcoming attempts to divide the world into 'us' and 'them' — on perceiving that the protection of the majority is intimately linked to the protection of the minority.

Ultimately, the struggle against AIDS can be carried out only through collective effort and solidarity. It depends on education and information, on developing adequate services to care for the ill, on counselling and support for the infected and on basic health care services for all. These efforts can only be successful, however, to the extent that they draw people in rather than reject and alienate. It is only by including, rather than excluding, the people most affected by AIDS, that information and services will reach those most in need. It is only by including, rather than excluding, that the very fabric of society can be preserved, and that we can truly begin to struggle against AIDS, rather than against people living with AIDS. How we respond to these challenges, in Brazil, as in the rest of the world, will ultimately write the history of the third epidemic.

Part 2

Sexual Culture, Social Representations and HIV Transmission

Chapter 4

'Within Four Walls': Brazilian Sexual Culture and HIV/AIDS

Richard Parker

Since its original classification as a distinct set of related diseases, Acquired Immunodeficiency Syndrome (AIDS) has emerged as one of the major health problems facing the international community. Despite significant advances during recent years in the identification of the Human Immunodeficiency Virus (HIV) and the understanding of other physiological aspects of HIV infection, the social epidemiology of AIDS has remained relatively obscure. Most research has focused on the United States and Western Europe, with little attention to the cultural differences that may influence different patterns of HIV transmission. Even when a cross-cultural perspective has been proposed, it has generally failed to take into account the culturally constituted practices that affect the spread of HIV/AIDS (see, in particular, the discussion in Chapter 1 of this volume).

As a first step in seeking to unravel at least some of the hidden assumptions that have shaped so much of our thinking about HIV and AIDS both at home and abroad, this chapter focuses on the social and cultural construction of sexual conduct in contemporary Brazil. In particular, drawing on long-term ethnographic research on what has been described as Brazilian sexual culture (see Parker, 1991), it suggests some of the limitations that may exist in the categories and classifications that have most frequently been used to think about the dynamics of HIV transmission (see also Chapters 1 and 2 in this volume). Perhaps even more important, focusing on the local meanings associated with sexual experience in Brazil, it points to the importance that a more detailed understanding of cross-cultural particularity and difference might have in the development of a more effective response to HIV/AIDS in the future.

AIDS in Brazil

Even by the mid-1980s alarmingly high numbers of AIDS cases had been reported in Brazil. At first, however, these cases were the focus of relatively little attention. Indeed, AIDS was seen by many Brazilians, heavily influenced by the representations of local news media, as little more than a rather peculiar disease affecting the gay community in the United States (see also Chapters 2 and 3 in this volume).

By October 1983 thirteen cases of AIDS and nine deaths had been confirmed in São Paulo, and cases were beginning to appear in other states as well. Over the course of the next year the situation declined further, and by April 1984 forty-three cases and twenty deaths had been confirmed in São Paulo alone, and some seventy cases had been identified throughout the country as a whole — principally among homosexual men. By now, however, the so-called 'victims' of the epidemic also included at least seven 'bisexual' men and two 'heterosexual' women.

By the beginning of 1985 at least one new case of AIDS was being registered every day, and four deaths were attributed to the disease per week. The greatest concentration of cases was found in the Rio de Janeiro and São Paulo metropolitan areas; however, at least one case was reported in virtually every Brazilian state. In only two months during 1985 more cases had been reported than in all of 1983. Whatever its place of origin, the disease could no longer be considered simply a foreign import — it had taken root in Brazil.

By 1985, then, AIDS was beginning to be recognized as a significant health problem in Brazil, and late in that year, with 462 reported cases and 224 confirmed deaths, Brazil moved into fourth place (behind the United States, France and Haiti) in the list of nations with the highest number of confirmed cases. By July 1986 the number of registered cases had climbed to 790 and the number of confirmed deaths to 406, moving Brazil ahead of both Haiti and France and placing it second only to the United States with the highest incidence of AIDS outside Africa.

Indeed, these statistics offered only a partial picture of the epidemic in Brazil. Like Haiti and the nations of central Africa, Brazil is a tropical country, and its citizens have long been familiar with a wide range of endemic diseases that manifest symptoms similar to those of AIDS. Economic hardship too often constrains people's ability to seek professional medical advice, and even those sufferers who seek such help may be misdiagnosed. In addition, despite important advances in the general quality of medical services in Brazil over the past decades, the severe economic problems currently facing the nation have unavoidably limited the development of an infrastructure capable of confronting major public health problems.

Besides the important material conditions that have limited a fuller understanding of the AIDS epidemic in Brazil, however, an additional difficulty lies in the conceptual model that has been used by both AIDS researchers and by Brazilian society more generally to understand and respond to the spread of the disease. This model, constructed on the basis of data from the United States and Western Europe, focused almost exclusively on the apparent homosexual and bisexual transmission of HIV (see Chapters 1 and 2 in this volume). The fact of the matter, however, is that the nature of this relationship between sexuality and AIDS in Brazil seems to have been largely taken for granted, rather than carefully examined (see also Parker, 1992). It is on this question of sexual life and its relation to AIDS that my own ethnographic research on Brazil can perhaps offer a number of insights.

Since 1982, I have been involved in the study of sexual ideology and the social and cultural construction of sexual meanings throughout Brazil (see, in particular, Parker, 1991). The nature of this project began to take shape during a preliminary field trip in July and August 1982, when I went to Rio de Janeiro to study Portuguese and to make arrangements for more extensive fieldwork the following year. Quite by chance, I lived in a rather run-down section of central Rio which served as a focus for lower-class street prostitution. Even with the fairly limited informant relationships that I was able to establish during this period (mostly with young people in their late teens and early 20s who were helping me learn the language), it was possible to make some enquiries about the nature of this underworld and to come away with a sense that it was different in a number of significant ways from anything comparable in my own society.

I returned to Rio for a longer stay in August 1983. Though my initial intention was not a study of sexuality but a historical and political examination of Brazilian *carnaval*, I found myself returning, almost unavoidably, to the question of sexual life in Brazil. The centrality of sexual meanings in the symbolism of *carnaval* was impossible to ignore. Indeed, the study of *carnaval* quickly became but one part of a much more inclusive study of the social and cultural construction of sexual ideology in urban Brazil.

This change of research focus was possible not merely because of the logical ties between the two subjects, but also because of the informant networks that I had begun to develop. During the first two months of my stay I lived in Catete, a middle- to lower-middle-class neighbourhood just south of the centre of Rio, and afterwards moved to a small apartment in the more well-to-do area of Copacabana. I did not focus my attention on the life of any particular community or neighbourhood, however, and concentrated instead on making contacts with men and women actively involved in preparations for *carnaval*. Focusing on the highly complex social networks related to the festival, I was thus brought into contact with a wide range of individuals — with *favelados* (shantytown dwellers), with members of the lower class, with members of the lower-middle and middle classes, and even with a few quite well-to-do men and women throughout Rio.

These same individuals served, at least initially, as my central informants not only about *carnaval* but also about the shape of Brazilian sexual culture. From roughly November 1983 to March 1984 I interviewed formally and informally the women and men whom I had met through these networks, seeking to uncover less the specifics of their own sexual lives than their understandings and interpretations of sexual life in Brazil more generally. During this period my informants were nearly equally divided along the lines of gender. They included most, if not all, of the sexual subtypes that we, in our own tradition, would be inclined to recognize: both female and male prostitutes, as well as their clients; self-identified lesbians and male homosexuals; male and female bisexuals; both single and married heterosexuals, with and without children; and so on. My informants also tended to be relatively young — almost all between 18 and 40 years of age. The work was entirely qualitative; I made no attempt to gather detailed statistical information or to conduct quantitative surveys. Indeed, given the sensitive nature of the subject matter, there is no doubt that whatever insights I might have gained were heavily dependent, for better or worse, on the quality of the relationships that I was able to develop with informants — as in any ethnographic work, on the mutual trust and friendship we were able to establish.

By March 1984 these varied contacts throughout metropolitan Rio had enabled me to form some notion of sexual life as it seemed to exist there — as well as of the class and status distinctions that seemed to affect it. In an attempt to broaden this view in a number of ways, I made short trips to São Paulo, Brasília, Salvador and Maceió, as well as to Recife and the interior of the state of Pernambuco, where I was able to spend time with the relatives of a number of my informants in Rio. Between March and July 1984 I split my time and activities between my base in Rio and a predominantly lower-class community situated on the outskirts of Petrópolis (a smaller city in the state of Rio de Janeiro), where I lived with the family of one of my closest informants in Rio. Here, within the context of a more clearly defined community, my friends and informants ranged from children of 9 or 10 to older individuals in their 60s and 70s. There I was able to get a view of family life that was far more intimate and more detailed than anything that I had been exposed to in Rio.

Through these diverse contacts I sought to examine the sometimes contradictory cultural patterns — the ideological constructs and the value systems — that work to shape the sexual universe in contemporary Brazil. I tried to extrapolate the underlying, and often unconscious, yet very much culturally constructed, rules that organize sexual life there — a cultural grammar, if you will, in which I think most Brazilians (and especially most urban Brazilians) are more or less competent and on which individuals draw to generate their own unique performances (see Parker, 1991).

During this 1983–84 study cases of AIDS were first reported in Brazil, and I returned to Rio and Petrópolis in July and August 1986 to focus specifically on that problem. It was then that I became convinced that it was necessary to understand the social and cultural construction of sexual life in Brazil before it would be possible to comprehend AIDS epidemiology there and take effective measures to combat the further spread of HIV infection.

Brazilian Sexual Culture

Sexual Classifications

The main categories that have dominated the discussion of AIDS internationally — 'heterosexuality' (*heterossexualidade*), 'homosexuality' (*homossexualidade*) and 'bisexuality' (*bissexualidade*) — are clearly present in Brazilian culture. Nonetheless, they have a history that is linked, as in Western Europe and the United States, to the emergence of modern medical science. First introduced into Brazilian culture only in the mid-twentieth century through the work of social hygienists, medical doctors and psychoanalysts whose thinking had been influenced by a series of developments in European psychology and sexology, this new system of sexual classification has become more widely disseminated in recent years through its increasing use on radio, television and in the press. It remains, however, in large measure an elite discourse that has thus far made only limited inroads into popular usage (see Fry, 1982; Fry and MacRae, 1983; Parker, 1985, 1989, 1991).

Just as categories such as *heterossexualidade* and *homossexualidade* have only gradually begun to take hold in Brazilian life, the notion of an *identidade homossexual* (homosexual identity) or a distinct homosexual community or gay ghetto (a social configuration that has been taken as central to the early manifestation of AIDS in Europe and the United States) is at least partially foreign to the Brazilian situation. Something that may loosely be described as a 'gay community' has taken root, as we shall see, in the larger, more modernized urban centres of south-eastern Brazil (see Altman, 1980; Fry and MacRae, 1983; Trevisan, 1986). However, its shape and structure display significant differences from European and North American counterparts. Like the sexual classifications imported by the medical establishment, it has necessarily taken a distinct form in response to the social and cultural context within which it has developed (see Parker, 1989).

The structure of sexual life in Brazil has traditionally been conceived in terms of a model focused on the relationship between sexual practices and gender roles — on the distinction between masculine *atividade* (activity) and feminine *passividade* (passivity) as central to the order of the sexual universe. It is along the lines of such perceived *atividade* and *passividade* that the distinctions between *macho* (male) and *fêmea* (female), *masculinidade* (masculinity) and *feminilidade* (femininity), and the like, have traditionally been organized in Brazil. In daily life, however, such conceptions have been constructed in an almost entirely informal fashion, less as the product of self-conscious reflection than of the popular language that Brazilians use to speak about and classify specific sexual practices (Parker, 1991).

The outlines of this cultural configuration emerge clearly in the language that Brazilians use to describe sexual relations — in their use of verbs, such as *comer* (to eat) and *dar* (to give), as metaphors for forms of sexual interaction. *Comer* describes the act of penetration during sexual intercourse. Used in a variety of contexts as a synonym for verbs such as *vencer* (to conquer, vanquish) and *possuir* (to posses, own), it implies a form of symbolic domination, as played out through sexual practice. In contrast, *dar* describes the role of being penetrated in either vaginal or anal intercourse. Just as *comer* suggests an act of domination, *dar* implies some form of submission or subjugation (Parker, 1991).

Drawing on these metaphors and using them as the basis for a set of classificatory categories, the sexual universe in Brazil can be structured along lines rather different from the distinction between *homossexualidade* and *heterossexualidade*. On the one hand, there are those who *comem*, who symbolically consume their partners by taking the active role during sexual intercourse, and, on the other hand, those who *dão*, who passively offer themselves to be penetrated and possessed by their active partners. Within this system of classification it is the first of these two groups that Brazilian culture defines — in view of their active, phallic domination — as *homens* or 'men' (Fry, 1982, 1985; Fry and MacRae, 1983; Parker, 1985, 1989, 1991).

If this first category seems rather straightforward, the second group, those who *dão*, is less so, as it includes not only the *mulher* or 'woman', but also a third figure known as the *viado* (from *veado* 'deer') or *bicha* (literally, 'worm, intestinal parasite', but also the feminine form of *bicho*, 'animal', and frequently explained by informants as a 'female animal') — terms that can perhaps be translated best as 'queer' or 'faggot'.[1] Although in fact biologically male in terms of anatomy, the *viado* or *bicha* is nonetheless linked to the *mulher* in terms of social role. Having adopted the fundamentally passive, feminine role of being penetrated in same-sex anal intercourse, the *viado* or *bicha* becomes a kind of symbolic equivalent of the biological female. Even as a kind of symbolic female, however, the *viado* or *bicha* remains, at least in terms of popular conception, something of a failure on both social and biological counts: not an *homem* because of unacceptably feminine behaviour, yet unable to play out the role of the *mulher* fully because of anatomy (see Altman, 1980; Fry, 1985; Parker, 1985, 1989, 1991; Young, 1973).[2]

The evaluative distinctions that are implicitly created in this popular set of classificatory categories stand in sharp contrast to the 'medical/scientific' notions of *homossexualidade* and *heterossexualidade*. For, while the *viado* or *bicha* suffers serious social stigma, the same is not so clearly true of his sexual partners. Within this more popular system of sexual classification, it is at least potentially possible for the *homem* to enter into sexual relations not only with *mulheres* but also with other biological males (the *viado* or *bicha*) without sacrificing his masculine identity. Precisely because his phallic dominance is preserved through his performance of the active role in sexual intercourse, the *masculinidade* of the *homem* is never fundamentally called into question, regardless of the biological sex of his partners. While the *homem* will no doubt be far less likely to flaunt his conquest of other males publicly, he is nonetheless reasonably free within the context of this system to pursue occasional or even ongoing sexual contacts with both males and females without fear of severe social sanction (see Fry, 1982, 1985; Fry and MacRae, 1983; Parker, 1985, 1989, 1991).[3]

What is perhaps most striking about this configuration is the fluidity of sexual desire that it suggests.[4] While the medical/scientific system of sexual classification seems to postulate a stable correspondence among desire, practice and identity, the Brazilian folk model would seem to imply a rather more flexible relationship among these components of an individual's sexual life.

It is largely because of the fundamental contrast between the folk and the medical/scientific models that the latter has taken only a very tentative hold of the Brazilian sexual landscape. Its influence has been limited almost entirely to the middle and upper classes in Brazil's larger, more modernized cities. Although the new terminology has become increasingly widespread (thanks largely to its dissemination through Brazil's growing mass media), it has remained at best superimposed on the older folk beliefs and classifications and appears to exercise virtually no influence over Brazilians living outside major urban centres. Even where it has exerted a certain impact in the cities and among the elite, the medical/scientific model has often been reinterpreted in traditional folk concepts, with their emphasis not on sexual object choice, as in the categories *homossexualidade* or *heterossexualidade*, but rather on *atividade* and *passividade*. In popular thought, the category of *homossexuais* or 'homosexuals' has most often been reserved for 'passive' partners, while the classification of 'active' partners in same-sex interactions has remained rather unclear and ambiguous.

While the influence of the medical/scientific system of sexual classification has been limited, it has not been entirely absent. It has for some time structured the ways in which a variety of social institutions — ranging from the police and the military to the medical establishment — have classified same-sex interactions (Fry and MacRae, 1983; Trevisan, 1986). It seems to have played an important role, as well, in fostering the development in Brazil during the late 1960s and 1970s both of something resembling an *identidade homossexual*, principally among members of the middles class, and of the gradual construction of a *comunidade gay* or 'gay community', modelled on the emerging gay subcultures of European and North American cities (Altman, 1980; Fry, 1982; Fry and MacRae, 1983; MacRae, 1990; Parker, 1989; Trevisan, 1986). While these developments have been quite consciously linked by Brazilians themselves to historical transformations taking place outside their country, they have nonetheless continued to respond to and reflect the traditional structure of sexual relations in Brazil, and can only be fully understood in relation to these structures.

The result of the interplay between traditional and modern models for sexual behaviour has been the construction of an open, shifting and flexible subculture of *entendidos* (those who know) in Brazil's larger cities. This subculture has been organized mainly around same-sex practices and desires, played out in such typical meeting places as bars, beaches, saunas, discos and the like. Central to this sexual subculture has been the development of a new category, the *entendido* (or *entendida* in the case of women). This category applies not only to those individuals who have adopted a strictly homosexual or gay identity, based on what they perceive as a more modern, North American or European model, but also to anyone who has been drawn to and takes part in this somewhat secretive underworld.[5] Though some *entendidos* choose to *se assumir* (roughly equivalent to the English notion, 'coming out'), most do not, and the public declaration of a homosexual identity has been limited mainly to middle-class participants in Brazil's small *movimento homossexual* or 'gay liberation movement'. This movement has failed to touch the lives of the vast majority of men and women who make up this loosely structured *entendido* subculture (Daniel and Míccolis, 1983; Fry and MacRae, 1983; Parker, 1989; Trevisan, 1986).

What has developed within this urban subculture is a further elaboration of sexual types, based principally on the active/passive distinction of popular culture but played out in variable same-sex desires and practices. Thus *entendidos* are sometimes contrasted with *homens*, with every implication that sexual interactions can and will take place between them. The traditional *bicha* is described as the passive partner of the active *bofe* — a term which is roughly equivalent to 'stud' in English, and is used to describe masculine *homens* who nonetheless take part principally in the subculture of the *entendidos*. The same kinds of distinctions have also been applied to the world of male prostitution, where a sharp line is drawn between the highly masculine *michê* or 'hustler' and the ambiguously feminine *travesti* or 'transvestite', both of whom are common, almost paradigmatic, figures in the (homo) sexual subcultures of most major urban centres in Brazil (see Chapter 5 in this volume). Indeed, the same dichotomy even structures the increasingly open presence of the once almost invisible *lésbica* or 'lesbian', classified more typically as the *sapatão* (literally, big shoe, but used much like the English notion of 'dyke' or 'butch dyke') and the *sapatilha* (literally, slipper, roughly equivalent to 'femme dyke').

This rather elaborate cast of characters has come to people the drama of sexual life in the homosexual subcultures of major Brazilian cities (and increasingly of the smaller cities as well). It is characterized by its flexibility and its fluidity. New players are constantly entering the scene, while others quietly depart. In addition, the cast of characters seems strikingly transformable, because the very distinctions that seem to organize life within this subculture can at any moment be overturned, undercut and rearranged. For the right price any client can succeed in *comendo* or 'eating' the *michê*; the married *homem* will just as likely *dá* or 'give' to the travesti; or the *travesti*, in turn, might even find herself involved in sexual relations with the *sapatão*. Indeed, it is central to this subculture — and, I believe, to Brazilian sexual ideology as a whole — that the categories that seem most fixed, most absolute, can always be transformed, and that the constancy of sexual classifications can be relativized and overcome in the reality of erotic practice (Parker, 1991).[6]

Erotic Practices

As socially and culturally constituted in Brazil — again, principally within the language of popular culture as opposed to the more limited discourses of various elites — erotic experience is centrally dependent upon at least two sets of interrelated distinctions or oppositions: a distinction between prohibition and transgression, on the one hand, and between public and private experience, on the other. That certain sexual acts should be culturally defined as permissible and others as prohibited should come as no great surprise. What is perhaps less easily understood, yet nonetheless crucial, is that from the Brazilian perspective the very notion of prohibition implies the equally culturally determined possibility of sexual transgression. The undermining in private of otherwise oppressive public norms is central to the meaning of erotic practice in Brazilian life (Parker, 1991).

The nature of the distinctions between prohibition and transgression and between public and private is captured with particular clarity in the language of daily life or popular culture. Expressions, such as '*Entre quatro paredes, tudo pode acontecer*' (Within four walls, everything can happen) or '*Por de baixo do pano, tudo pode acontecer*' (Beneath the sheets, everything can happen), can be used in a variety of contexts and are explained by Brazilians themselves as explicitly sexual in origin. While such expressions are subject to a good deal of variation in their exact wording, their underlying meaning remains unchanged: the notion of being somehow *escondido* or 'hidden', regardless of one's specific physical surroundings. Whether 'within four walls', 'beneath the sheets', or in any other situation in which one is somehow 'concealed' or even 'disguised', it is possible to encounter a freedom of sexual expression that would be explicitly prohibited in the 'outside', 'public' world. In the freedom of such private, hidden moments, Brazilians suggest, anything can happen, everything is possible (Parker, 1991).

The concept of *tudo* or 'everything' is central here; it is perhaps the key component in the domain that Brazilians call *sacanagem* (Da Matta, 1983; Parker, 1991). Much like the folk model of sexual actors, which tends to cut across region and class in Brazil, *sacanagem* is an extremely complex cultural category with no suitable English translation.[7] In the present context, however, it can be described roughly as the popular category which Brazilians use to label the world of erotic experience. Within this world, which is focused on private as opposed to public meanings, the significance of sexual practices takes shape less as an expression of an overriding system of sexual classification based on activity/passivity, sexual object choice and so on, than as an end in itself. It does not centre on one's identity, on some inner truth of the sexual self, but on *tesão* (sexual excitement) and *prazer* (pleasure). In *fazendo tudo* or 'doing everything' (i.e., precisely those practices which the public world most strictly circumscribes and prohibits), one most clearly embodies the erotic ideal of *sacanagem* (Da Matta, 1983; Parker, 1991).

This focus on the realization of momentary pleasures reinforces the fluidity of sexual desire that seems so evident in the classification of sexual actors and the construction of homosexual practices. The emphasis on *fazendo tudo* as fundamental to the fulfilment of both *tesão* and *prazer* places special emphasis on broadening one's repertoire of sexual practices as widely as possible. Thus rather elaborate and varied forms of sexual foreplay, a strong emphasis on oral sex, and especially a focus on anal intercourse, all take their place alongside vaginal intercourse as important elements in the cultural 'scripting' of erotic interactions (on sexual scripts, see Gagnon and Simon, 1973; Simon and Gagnon, 1984; see also Parker, 1991).

Learning the script for a variety of sexual acts is evident in the sexual explorations of young children and adolescents. For example, in the game *troca-troca* (literally, exchange-exchange) pubescent and adolescent boys take turns, each inserting his penis in the other's anus. In addition, the early sexual interactions of adolescent boys and girls draw on a wide range of non-vaginal sexual practices, in particular on anal intercourse, in order to avoid both unwanted pregnancy and rupture of the hymen (*cabaço*), still an important sign of a young woman's sexual purity. It is also widely acknowledged that both married and unmarried men turn to the services of prostitutes for the commonly cited reason that paid professionals perform a range of sexual acts that a proper wife and mother might shun (on prostitution in Brazil, see Fonseca, 1982; Freitas, 1985; Gaspar, 1985; Perlongher, 1987a).

What these ideas construct, in short, is an erotic universe focused on the transgression of public norms through a kind of playfulness reminiscent of *carnaval*. The transgressions that were part of one's adolescent sexual experience and the excitations they produced play themselves out again repeatedly throughout adult life. They undercut the effects of sexual prohibitions and make polymorphous pleasures, such as oral and anal intercourse, an important part even of married, heterosexual relationships. Such acts, along with the *tesão* or excitement which is thought to underlie them and the *prazer* or enjoyment which is understood to be their aim, are as much a product of the Brazilian cultural construction of reality as is the classification of sexual actors into *homens* and *mulheres; viados* or *bichas; heterossexuais, homossexuais* and *bissexuais; entendidos, bofes, michês, travestis, sapatões* and the like. Like such categories, this erotic ideology provides a framework that must be understood if we are to begin to make sense of the epidemiology and control of AIDS in Brazil.

Predicting the Future and Responding to the Epidemic

The cultural categories and ideas that map out the sexual universe in contemporary Brazil should not, of course, be confused with sexual behaviour itself, which is, after all, the way in which the HIV is most frequently transmitted. The social sciences have long recognized the often great discrepancy, and sometimes even contradiction, between ideological constructs and actual behaviours. Thanks to the detailed statistical work of Kinsey and his colleagues in the United States (Kinsey *et al.*, 1948, 1953), this discrepancy has certainly been confirmed in the area of sexual activity.[8]

Yet even among Kinsey's followers, the behavioural focus that dominated sex research during the 1940s and 1950s has given way to the understanding that sexual conduct, like any other form of human behaviour, is learned within society — that sexual behaviours are socially and culturally organized or scripted (see, in particular, Gagnon and Simon, 1973, Plummer, 1975, 1982; Weeks, 1981, 1985). To the extent that the cultural configurations that we have examined function, like other cultural systems, as models both of and for reality, then their influence on the lives that they touch, and in particular, their potential impact on the course of the AIDS epidemic, can hardly be ignored.

Indeed, for anyone familiar with the epidemiology of AIDS and the complex prevention and treatment issues it raises, the implications of the various dimensions of Brazilian sexual culture that we have reviewed will perhaps be evident. Yet it is worth articulating them as clearly as possible. In particular, I shall focus on the potential impact of this ideological configuration on three crucial, and obviously interrelated, areas of concern: (1) the transmission of HIV in the Brazilian population; (2) the education of the Brazilian public about AIDS and about the reduction of risk; and (3) the care and treatment of AIDS patients, including the organized, institutional response to related practical problems that have increasingly been posed by a growing epidemic.

HIV Transmission

Although HIV may have entered Brazil initially through a series of same-sex contacts and, particularly in the earliest years of the epidemic, remained closely linked to the homosexual subculture, the probability that this will continue to be the case seems highly remote. On the contrary, the polymorphous character of sexual desire and, in particular, the flexible structure of both homosexual practices and the homosexual subculture in Brazil make the categorization of homosexuals as a distinct 'high-risk' group rather questionable in the long run. I suggest that the epidemiological validity of this categorization will break down far more rapidly in Brazil than in either Europe or the United States. The multiple interconnections that seem to link *viados* to *homens*, *entendidos* to *michês*, *travestis* to *michês*, *entendidos* to *homens*, and ultimately *homens* to *mulheres* are too complex and intricate to warrant the simplistic view of sexual contact embodied in current epidemiological thinking. Indeed, it is worth noting in this regard that even by December 1986 more than 20 per cent of the AIDS patients being cared for at hospitals in Rio de Janeiro were classified (in terms, of course, of medical/ scientific categories) as *bissexuais* — a percentage as much as ten times greater than that registered at most hospitals in Western Europe and the United States (Costa, 1986).

This picture is complicated even further, I believe, by factors such as the widespread practice of anal intercourse between men and women. Anal intercourse is central to male same-sex interactions in Brazil, regardless of the specific sexual identities of the participants. Furthermore, as we have seen, in the developing gay communities of major cities participants in this form of intercourse are increasingly switching behavioural roles. In addition, anal intercourse appears to be a common practice in sexual interactions between males and female prostitutes and is also a part of the sexual life of many heterosexual couples. While there exists nothing for Brazil even remotely comparable to the Kinsey studies that might be used to substantiate the frequency of these practices, a recent piece of research is worth noting. Based on 5000 interviews of men and women throughout the nation, the study found that over 50 per cent of those interviewed in Rio de Janeiro and over

40 per cent of those interviewed in the rest of Brazil reported practising anal intercourse at least occasionally (Santa Inez, 1983).

Since unprotected anal intercourse has been singled out as a major vehicle for transmission of HIV (see, for example, Johnson and Vieira, 1986), these cultural and behavioural data gain particular importance for the epidemiology of the disease in Brazil. Although there is a good deal of debate concerning the relative efficiency of HIV transmission in relation to different sexual practices, it seems clear that the mucus of the anus may be less resistant to friction than that of the vagina, and that microscopic tears occur during anal intercourse which permit direct entry of semen into the bloodstream. Since anal intercourse has thus been identified as an especially efficient mode of HIV transmission, the apparently frequent practice of anal sex not only between men but also between women and men in Brazil thus makes the epidemiological picture for AIDS there quite distinct from the picture in Europe and the United States. Specifically, patterns of anal intercourse significantly change the definition of 'high-risk groups' in Brazil and may well further the spread of HIV and AIDS within the population at large.

Public Education about AIDS

With the hope of an effective vaccine still unfulfilled, public education and the use of safer sexual practices have proven to be the most effective means of limiting the spread of HIV transmission in both the United States and Western Europe. Because of inadequate governmental support and funding for such measures, however, even in the US and Europe, their effectiveness has depended in large part upon the pre-existence of a distinct gay community with developed medical and journalistic institutions that are capable of reaching both a self-identified homosexual audience (the 'high-risk' group), as well as a wider audience outside that bounded community. The information made available through such institutions has influenced sexual practices only because of the gradual development of a sense of risk on the part of the public and a subsequent willingness to transform the shape and structure of erotic practices in response to the perceived risk (see, for example, Patton, 1985; Pollak, 1988).

In Brazil, although there does exist a distinct subculture organized around same-sex desires and practices, there is little in the way of a well organized homosexual community with its own institutions and publications. While 'safe sex' pamphlets have been published by gay groups and AIDS organizations in Brazil, their impact has been limited. Such materials have generally been oriented toward a rather limited group with a homosexual identity (*identidade homossexual*), rather than toward the much wider population engaged in behaviours that are considered to pose especially high risk of transmission. This lack of sensitivity to the reality of Brazilian sexual culture has also been manifest in the publication of informational pamphlets that are direct translations of information distributed to the public in the United States. Indeed, the very notion of 'safe sex' found in much educational material, which often focuses on restricting the sexual repertoire, runs directly counter to the Brazilian emphasis on *fazendo tudo*, with all its excitingly dangerous connotations. Ultimately, it seems impossible to expect significant results in Brazil from educational materials that are oriented toward sexual identity rather than behaviour and that ignore the role of culture in constituting erotically satisfying and meaningful experience.

Yet perhaps nothing so seriously limits the potential impact that even the most culturally sensitive campaign for safer sex practices might have in Brazil so much as the continued denial on the part of the vast majority of Brazilians (regardless of their sexual orientation or activities) of the danger posed to them as individuals by the spread of AIDS. This issue of denial, I suspect, is the crucial one facing both individual Brazilians and Brazilian society as a whole in seeking to grapple with the problems posed by AIDS. Even though the epidemiological facts would suggest a different response, Brazilians in the main have accepted the overly simplistic characterization of the disease that has been imported from abroad and imposed uncritically on the Brazilian reality. Men involved in same-sex sexual practices, regardless of the ways in which they identify themselves as sexual beings, have focused on the characterization of AIDS as a disease of the developed world and have written off its potential danger through any number of explanations. Some of my own informants have suggested that Brazilian blood will prove unusually resistant to the virus. Others have suggested that careful hygiene following sexual intercourse will be the key to continued health. Still others have argued that the effects of AIDS have been exaggerated as part of a moralistic attack against gays in Brazilian society (for comparable arguments, see, for example, the discussions in *Veja*, 1985a: 66–67).

If individuals involved in same-sex practices have generally sought to deny the specific risks of AIDS for Brazilians, those not involved in such practices, or involved in only limited ways, have largely sought to deny the danger that the disease poses to them personally by viewing it as a *praga gay* or 'gay plague', affecting only the homosexual population (with the referent of 'homosexual' left entirely unspecified). This perception has been reinforced in a number of ways. For example, medical authorities have irresponsibly disseminated untrue information about the disease at the same time as they have called for the reduction of civil liberties for homosexuals (see Trevisan, 1986). Reports in the popular news media have also characterized the epidemic sensationally and belittled its importance as a public health problem in Brazil (Daniel and Parker, 1991, as well as Chapter 3 in this volume; see also Trevisan, 1986). These forms of denial have resulted in an absolute distinction between 'self' and 'other', 'us' and 'them'. Playing upon the prejudices and stigmas already present in Brazilian society, they ignore the potential impact that AIDS almost surely will have on the Brazilian population more generally.

AIDS Treatment

Locating notions of disease and contagion in concrete persons opens the way for any number of cruelties and inhumanities. Specific instances in Brazil, as in other parts of the world, are all too easy to cite, and have already been documented in some detail elsewhere (see, in particular, Chapters 2 and 3 in this volume). Yet as disturbing as each individual case of inhumanity clearly is, they pale in comparison with the prospective problems of handling the epidemic toward which Brazil may well be headed and against which the Brazilian authorities seem to have taken few steps to respond. Both the Brazilian government and the medical community in the private sector (with a few significant exceptions — e.g., *Jornal do Brasil*, 1987) have consistently tended to downplay the public health danger of AIDS in Brazil. In the words of Carlos Sant'Anna, who served as the Brazilian Minister of Health until February 1986, in responding to AIDS, 'we are discussing a disease which is preoccupying, but not a priority' (see *New York Times*, 1985, 1986; *Veja*, 1985a: 56). It must be acknowledged that, from Sant'Anna's perspective, such a statement is perhaps understandable. Officials who administer health programs for a nation that already suffers the effects of epidemic and endemic diseases may well consider reported cases of AIDS as relatively insignificant.

In spite of the immensity of the national health problem overall, a number of important steps have been taken to combat AIDS. In 1985 and 1986 a *Programa Nacional de Combate à AIDS* (National Program to Combat AIDS) was launched to bring together AIDS researchers, monitor the spread of the HIV infection, organize treatment services and educate the public (*Jornal do Brasil*, 1986; see also Chapter 1 in this volume). Plans for further educational programs and obligatory screening of the supplies of all blood banks have been developed, and national legislation banning discrimination against people with AIDS has been planned (*New York Times*, 1986; *Jornal do Brasil*, 1986). Yet the resources provided by the Ministry of Health to the *Programa Nacional* have generally fallen far short of the perceived need (see, for example, *Jornal do Brasil*, 1986). Some private hospitals still refuse to accept AIDS patients, and the government-operated university hospitals, which have treated most patients, are already greatly overtaxed. As the situation currently stands, the spread of HIV infection and AIDS continues unabated, and is likely to continue so for some time in the future.

Conclusions

The arguments developed here are necessarily tentative. Though the cultural outlines seem clear, their behavioural correlates are not. In part, this is because of the inherent difficulty in acquiring accurate data on sexual practices. Yet efforts to collect these data in terms of the categories of Brazilian sexual culture have been virtually non-existent. Even if tentative, however, the findings of this research, which has focused precisely on the aspects of Brazilian sexual culture that have previously been ignored, raise a number of important practical and conceptual issues. Specifically, they carry implications for public health in Brazil, for the understanding of AIDS in cross-cultural perspective, and more broadly for the role of cultural analysis in epidemiological research on such significant health problems as HIV/AIDS.

Most immediately, it is clear that a careful examination of the cultural context in Brazil inevitably leads to the conclusion that the health problem posed by AIDS and facing Brazilian society is potentially far more widespread and serious than has thus far been acknowledged. No less important, the actions being taken in response to the epidemic are inadequate in relation to the potential crisis at hand. Brazil is facing an epidemic disease that is potentially as devastating as any of the other serious public health problems that already exist there, and a combination of prejudice, short-sighted planning and economic instability has left Brazilian society almost entirely unprepared to confront it. Changes in both official and popular attitudes toward AIDS must be made, and they must be made rapidly.

In addition to increasing awareness of the potential health problems posed for Brazil by the spread of HIV/AIDS, the cultural data described in this chapter reveal several significant features of the

Brazilian case that are not incorporated into the dominant models that have been developed to describe the manifestations of AIDS internationally. These differences must be taken into account in seeking to build up a more complete understanding of AIDS as a cross-cultural phenomenon. It is tempting to suggest Brazil as a potential third model that might be added to the cases of the industrialized West and the central African nations in broadening our understanding of AIDS. Beyond simply adding another model, however, my hope is that a careful examination of the Brazilian case might help to deconstruct existing models. In short, the Brazilian alternative may help us to analyze the models themselves not as objective, scientific reality, but as cultural constructs.

Deconstructing these disease models, in turn, should lead us in a number of important (and interrelated) directions. Perhaps foremost, it should push us toward ever more detailed examinations of specific examples, such as Brazil, in seeking to understand the manifestations of AIDS within the range of social and cultural contexts. Such studies, drawing, as they must, on indigenous categories and classifications, might then enable us to build a wider understanding of AIDS based more on the detailed interpretation of cross-cultural differences (as well as similarities) than on the preconceived notions of Western medical science. It is imperative, given the international dimensions of the AIDS epidemic, that generalizable models of the disease be constructed in order to help combat it more effectively. As in all sound cross-cultural research, however, the road to the general may lie through attention to the particular (Geertz, 1973). Thus, through a rapid increase in both the number and sophistication of specific studies of AIDS in particular settings, one can more readily construct the broader explanatory and intervention models that are needed.

Finally, an awareness of the contribution that cultural analysis can make to epidemiological research on AIDS should lead us ultimately to appreciate diseases as both sociocultural and biological phenomena. Precisely because AIDS is a disease that links sickness to sexuality, it is simultaneously a sociocultural and a biological phenomenon. To understand AIDS and to struggle against it, then, we must ultimately confront it as much in sociocultural as in biomedical terms.

Notes

1 There is a good deal of historical and regional variation in the terminology, but labels such as *viado* and *bicha* were the terms most commonly used by

my own informants in the field. The reasons given for this selection varied. The frailness of the deer and, in more than one instance, of Walt Disney's creation, 'Bambi', in particular, was frequently cited as important to the choice of *viado*. The importance of effeminacy was clearly cited in the definition of *bicha* as well, with most informants explaining the term, as I have noted, as signifying some kind of indeterminate, and thus fundamentally anomalous, female animal. At least one informant suggested derivation from the French *biche* or 'doe', and thus neatly linked the notions of 'deer' and 'female animal'.

2 This emphasis on a distinction between activity and passivity in the structure of same-sex relationships is quite widespread. For similar constructs in other parts of Latin America, see, for example, Carrier, 1985; Lancaster, 1986; Taylor, 1985.

3 I suspect that *homens* are not more open about their experiences with *viados* in large part because of the continued presence of the Catholic moral code, which — however relaxed it may seem to be in Brazil — still explicitly condemns acts of *sodomia* (sodomy).

4 For a helpful discussions of the notion of 'fluidity' as it applies to sexual identity, see Herdt, 1984. On sexual desire, sexual practice and sexual identity as crucial issues in any discussion of sexuality, see Patton, 1985. On the social and cultural construction of sexual reality more generally, see Weeks, 1985.

5 The distinctions here are especially difficult to grasp, as they are both similar to, yet different from, our own. In the past both Peter Fry and I have suggested that the notion of the *entendido* could be understood as roughly parallel to the notion of the 'gay person' in the industrialized West — that it was imported to Brazil during the 1970s principally by members of the middle class who had adopted a 'homosexual identity', modelled along the lines being developed in the gay communities of the United States and Western Europe (Fry, 1982; Parker, 1985). This impression is strengthened by the fact that the term *gay* (which is also occasionally written as *guei*) was brought into Brazilian Portuguese at much the same time. The term *gay*, however, was quickly reinterpreted. Its meaning shifted dramatically from English usage, and it has come to be applied often to the most effeminate members of the homosexual subculture in Brazil. *Entendido*, on the other hand, has had a broader usage. Fry now believes that it was employed well before the emergence of a gay community in North America or Europe in order to refer to anyone who knew about and took part in same-sex interactions, as well as the subculture organized around these interactions (personal communication). It continues, as I understand it, to refer to individuals who consciously view themselves as *homossexuais*, as well as to individuals who do not hold a strictly homosexual self-image, but who engage from time to time in same-sex sexual practices.

6 In speaking of a 'Brazilian sexual ideology', I do not mean to suggest that the sexual experience of all Brazilians is somehow fundamentally the same

— that all Brazilians share the same sexual character. Even in a context less diverse than Brazil, such an assertion would seem unlikely. My argument is that sexual diversity among Brazilians is made possible by an ideological context that most Brazilians do in fact share. My interest is thus not simply the particular, and necessarily various, sexual realities of different Brazilians from whatever specific region or class, but the wider cultural patterns which quite literally make possible and help to structure such diversity throughout Brazil.

7 *Sacanagem* carries a variety of meanings that seem rather distant from its sexual connotations, but which tie into a common underlying theme. It can refer, for instance, to the experience of small injustices — much as we speak in English of have been 'screwed over' or 'fucked over' by someone or something. It can be used more playfully, as well, to describe the friendly teasing of one's fellows. In each of these instances, as well as in its more direct reference to the sex act, *sacanagem* possesses a certain rebellious quality — it refers to some form of transgression, a breaking of the rules of proper decorum and a denial of some form of social prohibition (see Parker, 1991).

8 As I have already noted, no adequate statistical studies of sexual practices have been carried out in Brazil. The few attempts that have been made to gather these data have invariably been by doctors and scientists, who have framed their questions in the language of the medical/scientific model rather than in the language of popular culture. See, for example, Santa Inez, 1983.

Chapter 5

The Negotiation of Difference: Male Prostitution, Bisexual Behaviour and HIV Transmission

Richard Parker

Although the role of prostitution in the transmission of HIV has been extensively debated over a number of years now, relatively little is known about what prostitution entails in different social and cultural settings (de Zalduondo, 1991). While research on prostitution and AIDS has become increasingly extensive in both epidemiology and social science, the behavioural links between sex work and HIV have often been more assumed than understood, and the social and cultural construction of prostitution has generally received less attention than the perceived threat supposedly posed by prostitutes to an unsuspecting public (Alexander, 1987). Assessment of the risks of HIV transmission within the sex industry, and even interventions aimed at responding to these risks, have rarely been founded on a full understanding of the specific behaviours involved or the social, cultural, economic and political forces that ultimately shape these behaviours and condition both the perception of risk and the possibility of risk reduction.

If a relative lack of understanding has characterized the discussion of prostitution generally, however, it has perhaps been even more pronounced in the case of male prostitution than in that of female prostitution. Indeed, even the increasing research attention that has been directed to the sex industry has largely failed to include male prostitution as an important research topic, and the widespread concern that sex work may be an important vector of HIV infection to a wider public has rarely been raised in relation to the practice of male prostitution (presumed principally to touch the lives of an already clearly defined 'risk group' rather than the 'general public'). Less visible, less clearly organized and no doubt less statistically significant than female prostitution, male prostitution has thus been, if anything, even less understood than female prostitution; and the social and cultural construction of male prostitution in specific settings has largely been ignored in what is an even more limited research literature (see Robinson, 1989).

This chapter aims to fill at least some of the gaps in our understanding of HIV transmission by focusing on the social and cultural construction of male prostitution in Brazil. Drawing on ethnographic research carried out over a number of years principally in Rio de Janeiro, it focuses on the diverse forms that male prostitution actually takes, even in a single site, suggesting that male prostitution (like female prostitution) is a more complex and diverse phenomenon than has generally been recognized. Examining the specific sexual behaviours that link male prostitutes not only to clients but also to non-commercial sexual partners, it suggests that the risks of HIV transmission raised by the practice of prostitution are very real, but that they can be defined and understood in far more specific terms than has thus far been the case in the generally vague discussions of much epidemiological and medical literature. Finally, drawing on this understanding, it examines some of the implications that detailed ethnographic description might have for the design and implementation of interventions aimed at reducing the risk of HIV infection.[1]

Male Prostitution and HIV Infection in Brazil

Perhaps the most basic point that must be made in seeking to understand prostitution generally, and male prostitution in particular, is that the phenomenon of prostitution is in no way uniform or singular. At its most minimal, the definition of prostitution as the exchange of sexual services for money, gifts, favours or what have you, actually obscures not only significant cross-cultural differences, but also the no less important diversity that generally exists in any given social and cultural setting. Anywhere where one looks at the social construction of prostitution with any care, what will be found is not a single, unified behavioural construct, but a range of different behaviours — distinct forms of prostitution.

While this diversity in the construction of prostitution is evident in almost all social and cultural contexts, it is especially apparent in contemporary Brazil, where historical, cultural and economic forces have led to the perhaps unusually extensive elaboration of different forms of sex work — diverse types of prostitution that must be understood as part of a wider system. Distinctions can be made in differentiating, for example, lower income from higher income sex work, street prostitution from prostitution in houses, saunas or escort services and so on. Class, in particular, functions within Brazilian society as a key axis along which, or in terms of which, distinct forms of sex work can be distinguished and analyzed, with *prostituição de baixa renda* (low income prostitution) contrasted to *alta prostitutição* (high class prostitution).[2]

Yet it is perhaps gender, even more than class, that is central in seeking to understand the relationship between prostitution and HIV transmission in Brazil. Both male and female prostitution can be found in virtually all major urban areas. Throughout Brazil, however, a further distinction must also be made, within the context of what has been described as male prostitution, between the prostitution of *michês* or 'hustlers' and *travestis* or 'transvestites'.[3] Indeed, within the context of contemporary Brazilian culture, transvestite prostitution is so conceptually and behaviourally distinct that it should perhaps be situated between female prostitution and the male prostitution of *michês*, as a specific social and cultural construct in which both gender and sexuality are mapped out and performed in highly particular ways (Parker, 1988, 1989; see also Chapter 4 in this volume).

These distinctions have taken on particular importance, in turn, with the emerging AIDS epidemic. Limited seroprevalence studies have pointed to a relatively wide range of HIV infection levels among female sex workers in different urban centres, as well as among different subgroups within the same area, and have contributed to alarm about the risks posed by the practice of prostitution for the spread of HIV within the Brazilian population. In Brazil, as elsewhere, female prostitutes have thus often been scapegoated for the spread of AIDS to the wider, heterosexual public (Alexander, 1987; see also Chapter 3 in this volume). Perhaps as a reflection of the higher seroprevalence rates found among men who have sex with men, however, far greater incidence of HIV infection has consistently been found in studies of male and transvestite prostitutes than have thus far been registered among female sex workers, particularly in major urban centres such as Rio de Janeiro and São Paulo (see, for example, Cortes *et al.*, 1989a, 1989b, 1989c, 1989d). Although based on limited samples, seroprevalence rates ranging from 33 to 43 per cent have been found in tests of male prostitutes in Rio de Janeiro, for example, while rates as high as 64 per cent have been found among *travestis* in São Paulo (Cortes *et al.*, 1989b, 1989c; Suleiman *et al.*, 1989).

For a variety of reasons, the levels of HIV seroprevalence that have begun to emerge among both male and transvestite prostitutes in Brazil are especially worrisome. While it is impossible to calculate accurately the number of individuals involved, it is clear that prostitution offers one of the few viable economic options open to many individuals in contemporary Brazilian life (and the relatively large transvestite population, in particular, has few other alternatives in the Brazilian economy). The risks involved, not only for prostitutes and their clients, but for non-commercial sexual partners as well, touch the lives of relatively large numbers of people, and may pose a far more volatile threat of HIV transmission in Brazil (even among the so-called general population) than is the case, for example, with female prostitution. Yet the dynamics of transmission within these groups are still very poorly understood; and this lack of understanding is itself a reflection of the relatively limited understanding that the medical and scientific community has of sexual behaviour within these groups.

To even begin to understand the meaning of HIV seroprevalence rates among male and transvestite prostitutes, and to interpret the implications of seroprevalence for HIV transmission, then, it is necessary to situate these data within a wider context: to interpret them in relation to the social and cultural construction of sexual practice in contemporary Brazilian life. Within this wider context the sexual conduct of *michês*, *travestis* and their various sexual partners takes shape as part of a highly specific configuration of sexual meanings and behaviours in which many of the most commonly held assumptions about the nature of sexuality seem to dissolve or disappear. Situated within this context, however, it becomes possible to understand the specific behaviours involved in male prostitution in ways that offer new insight into patterns of HIV transmission as well as potential strategies for interventions aimed at risk reduction.

The Social Construction of Sexual Practice

This distinction between *michês* and *travestis* is itself a reflection of the social and cultural construction of homosexuality in Brazil. As has already been discussed (see, in particular, Chapters 1 and 4 in this volume), medical/scientific categories such as 'homosexuality' or 'heterosexuality' have traditionally been less important in Brazilian sexual culture than notions of 'activity' or 'passivity'. Linked, respectively, to culturally constituted conceptions of masculinity and femininity, this distinction between activity and passivity has continued to play a key role in structuring sexual practice in contemporary Brazilian life, and this is as true in same-sex interactions as it is in interactions with members of the opposite sex (see Fry, 1982; Fry and MacRae, 1983; Parker, 1985, 1989, 1991, as well as Chapters 1 and 4 in this volume).

Within this particular configuration of the sexual universe, then, the social construction of sexual meanings (and, by extension, of sexual relationships) has been marked by a relatively high degree of fluidity or flexibility (see Chapter 4 in this volume). A distinct sexual subculture focused on and organized around same-sex interactions has gradually taken shape and become increasingly visible in large cities such as Rio de Janeiro and Sao Paulo over a number of decades (Parker, 1989; Perlongher, 1987a; Trevisan, 1986). The boundaries of this subculture have been relatively open-ended, however, and it has been organized less around a shared sense of sexual identity than around a wide range of same-sex desires and practices (Parker, 1989). Indeed, it is characterized less by uniformity than by diversity, and is perhaps most visible not in terms of the groups or organizations that represent it, or even the social institutions that it has produced, than in terms of the sexual geography of the city — the specific territories where a range of different desires and practices is offered and sought (see Fry and MacRae, 1983; MacRae, 1987; Parker, 1989; Perlongher, 1987a).[4]

Male prostitution in Brazil, like other forms of sexual interaction between men, has taken shape within this urban subculture, and has reflected its basic patterns of organization and its extensive diversity. Perhaps nowhere is this more evident than in the sharp distinction drawn between *michês* and *travestis* — a distinction translated not only into a set of distinct behavioural patterns, but into a highly specific organization of geographic space and cultural meaning. While the *michês* are built up as hypermasculine figures who are stereotypically believed to perform the active role with their homosexually identified clients, the *travestis* are marked by an exaggerated femininity that is thought to be played out most clearly in their sexual passivity (see Chapter 4 in this volume). This most basic distinction, in turn, is transformed into diverse patterns that link *michês* and *travestis* to both their clients and their non-commercial sexual partners, as well as distinct territories and forms of organization within the wider sexual geography of the city (see, in particular, Perlongher, 1987a).

The *michês*, for example, in most major urban centres, are drawn from the lower sectors of society — from the poor *subúrbios* or 'suburbs' that lie in the outskirts of major urban centres such as Rio or São Paulo. They are generally young, adolescents, between the ages of 13 or 14 and 19 or 20, who ride the trains into the centre of the city and work, often sporadically, in a range of different streets or plazas known to offer sexual interactions with older, more well-to-do men who are willing to pay for sexual services. Depending on the specific setting, the negotiations involved may take diverse forms. In Rio, for example, there is the Praça Floriano in Cinelândia, where both *michês* and their *fregueses* or 'clients' take up posts on park benches and converse at some length before coming to an accord and leaving the plaza for any one of the inexpensive hotels for men that can be found nearby. Only a few minutes away, in Via Appia, an abandoned area that functions as a garbage disposal by day, the *michês* take up their positions in the shadows beneath trees or next to lamp posts, striking a pose or slowly masturbating themselves in view of their clients, who pass by in automobiles, stopping to negotiate before moving on to a home or apartment, a hotel or motel, or some more secluded spot where sexual activity can take place without the threat of interruption.[5]

As in other forms of prostitution, the negotiation between the *michê* and his client is a complex interaction in which both the price charged and the specific sexual practices involved must be specified. The question of sexual practice is crucial precisely because of the meanings associated with activity and passivity, since practices such as fellating another male or being anally penetrated by a client are highly problematic behaviours that implicitly call into question masculine identity, and are therefore rejected outright by a large number of *michês*. While others may be willing to negotiate such practices (and popular wisdom on the streets suggests that almost all the *michês* may at some point, in private settings, eventually engage at least occasionally in passive anal intercourse), an idealized pattern of active/passive distinctions is nonetheless constructed within this world, as the expected activity of the *michê* is contrasted with the passivity of his *maricona* (effeminate) clients. The *michê*'s active anal penetration of his clients thus becomes a kind of norm—a norm that can be, and often is, broken in practice, but that structures the nature of interactions and exchanges.

This emphasis on exaggerated masculinity and sexual activity is in many ways a logical necessity precisely because the prostitution of the *michês* is generally a relatively limited part of their lives. While they may work the streets a few nights a week, or even quite regularly during certain hours of the night and early morning, the vast majority of the *michês* continue to live with their families, or in the traditional neighbourhoods of their families, to maintain ongoing social relationships and participate in social networks within such conventional settings, and to engage in (hetero)sexual interactions with partners who know nothing of their involvement in male prostitution. Sexual activity in their work as *michês* appears, for many, to serve as a psychological defence, necessary to guarantee that their homosexual relations, performed in exchange for money or other material benefits, need not in any way call into question the terms of their heterosexual experience and masculine identity within a society that structures almost all sexual exchanges in terms of a rigorous hierarchy. Indeed, within the terms of this construction, turning a trick on Friday night may be the only way to assure the money necessary to take a girlfriend out on Saturday, and a series of relatively rigid social, cultural and psychological mechanisms is thus brought into play to ensure that these universes of experience never interpenetrate or mix.

While many of the same cultural patterns are clearly central, the prostitution of *michês* contrasts sharply with the prostitution of *travestis*. Like the majority of the *michês*, the *travestis* tend to be drawn almost exclusively from the poorest segments of Brazilian society. Except in some of the most marginalized *favelas*, however, the *travesti* is rarely tolerated in the poorer, more traditional suburban neighbourhoods that are frequently the home of the *michê*. On the contrary, in beginning to cross the lines of gender, the *travesti* has almost no choice but to leave behind family and friends in moving to the centre of cities such as Rio and São Paulo, where a mixture of socially marginal and often illegal activities creates not only a kind of moral region but a moral anonymity in which the traditional values of Brazilian society cease to function. Within this world (which is also the world of female prostitution, drug trafficking, homosexuality and, we should add, the more sporadic prostitution of the *michês*), given pervasive prejudice and discrimination, almost no options other than prostitution are open to the *travesti* for earning a living; as a result, almost all *travestis* quickly become involved in prostitution as their primary activity.

Ironically, in spite of this pervasive discrimination, an extensive market exists for the sexual services offered by the *travesti*. Again, at least at first glance, these sexual interactions would seem to be constructed in almost the opposite terms as those of the *michê*, with exaggerated emphasis placed upon the *travesti*'s sexual passivity and symbolic femininity. As in the case of the *michê*, however, things are not quite as simple as they might at first appear, and the *travesti*'s sexual interactions can often be complex. While many lower-class or more self-consciously masculine clients (described within this universe as *bofes* or 'studs') tend to request that the *travesti* take the passive role in anal intercourse, another market exists, particularly among more middle-class clients, in which, again at the client's request, the *travesti* assumes the active role. Indeed, these differences are elaborate enough that distinct territories are marked out for active or passive preferences, and *travestis* will even choose their areas of work on the basis of their disposition for one or the other role. In Rio, for example, *travestis* pre-ferring the passive role in anal intercourse can be found, in particular, in the area surrounding the Quinta de Boa Vista, a large park in the north of the city where a predominantly lower-class clientele can be found. Those who are willing to vary their sexual performances, or to take a more active role, may choose the central area of Lapa or the southern neighbourhoods of Gloria or Copacabana, where more middle-class clients are found who often prefer passive anal intercourse with their *travesti* partners.[6]

As in the case of the *michê*, specific practices (as well as prices) will need to be negotiated in all of these different settings, but the negotiation responds to a distinct set of rules and expectations. In spite of these variations, however, few of the *travesti*'s clients consider themselves to be engaging in homosexual behaviour, even when taking the passive role in anal intercourse, as the classification of the *travesti* as a kind of symbolic female is apparently sufficient to counteract even the most apparent contradictions involved in the intricacies of sexual practice. Almost all of the clients, regardless of the preferences that they exhibit in their interactions with *travestis*, are otherwise involved with female sexual partners as well (see Pinel, 1989).

Cut off from the family and friends that provide the most basic frame of social reference for the *michê*, *travestis* often live together sharing apartments or renting bed spaces in the centre of the city or in neighbourhoods (such as Copacabana in Rio) known to tolerate both sexual difference and prostitution.[7] They are perhaps less likely to be involved in ongoing relationships with non-commercial sexual partners than are the *michês*, but even this is far from absolute, and many *travestis* pass through periods of reasonably stable relationships. These non-paying partners are normally members of the popular sectors of Brazilian society, often themselves marginal in some way — involved as managers or middle men in female prostitution, participants in drug trafficking or some other illegal activity, or without work and willing to take advantage of the *travestis*' earnings. Like the *travestis*' clients, many (if not most) are sexually active, as well, with women. Few, however, consider themselves to be homosexual because of their interactions with the *travestis*, and active penetration of the *travesti* is by far the most common form of sexual interaction in these non-commercial interactions.

Ultimately, then, the prostitution of *michês* and the prostitution of *travestis* take shape, in their social organization and construction, as almost mirror images of one another — yet mirror images that are, ironically, constituted within precisely the same system of cultural meanings, in terms of the same cultural grammar. They form part of the wider sexual subculture focused on sex between men in contemporary Brazilian life, occupying their own particular territories within its specific sexual geography. Perhaps most important, however, at least in relation to HIV transmission and AIDS in Brazil, they offer among the clearest examples of the ways in which this diverse subculture is often less bounded and distinct than open and fluid. Precisely because of the ways in which sexual meanings are shaped within this world, the possibilities for bisexual behaviour consistently break down the barriers between homosexuality and heterosexuality in ways that have important implications for the spread of HIV and AIDS in Brazilian society. Nowhere is this more clearly evident than in the world of male prostitution, where the crossing of sexual boundaries (in a variety of different directions) is central to the social and cultural organization of sexual practice.

HIV Transmission and AIDS Prevention

While the picture that emerges here is obviously painted in relatively broad strokes, the key point is that a number of distinct forms of male prostitution have taken shape in contemporary Brazilian life — and that these diverse forms of prostitution very probably open up the risk of HIV infection in a number of different ways. As much in the prostitution of *travestis* as in the prostitution of *michês*, HIV transmission may ultimately be linked not only to homosexual, but to bisexual and even heterosexual contact, in a chain of sexual interactions that may pass through acts of prostitution, but that are by no means limited to or exclusively focused on such exchanges. In these different forms of interaction, however, the culturally structured character of sexual contact creates relatively distinct patterns of behaviour that must themselves be understood in order to understand the chain of HIV transmission.

In the case of the *michê*, for example, bisexual behaviour is most pronounced on the part of the prostitute himself, and opens up important risks not only for him but for his non-commercial sexual partners as well.[8] In the case of the *travesti*, on the contrary, bisexual behaviour is relatively rare (though not altogether unknown) on the part of the prostitute, but is quite common on the part of both commercial and non-commercial partners. Within the construction of these different forms of prostitution, then, the direction of HIV transmission, and its link to homosexual and heterosexual contact, may ultimately follow quite different patterns — patterns that are not simply random, but that obey a very clearly articulated cultural grammar.

Perhaps as important as the structure of sexual behaviours (that open up the concrete risk of HIV transmission) is the way in which these same cultural patterns may ultimately shape the perception of risk in quite specific ways for the various participants in different forms of male prostitution. Given the complex and often contradictory classification of sexual interaction depending on the perspective of different participants, the diverse individuals involved in commercial sex may have highly inconsistent notions of risk in their own lives. While some (like many of the homosexually identified clients of the *michê*) may perceive themselves to be at risk in their interactions, others (such as the heterosexually identified clients of the *travesti*) may not. Even when the question of risk is raised in relation to commercial interactions, it may quickly give way in non-commercial interactions: while a *michê* may be concerned about the risks posed through his homosexual contact with commercial partners, this same concern may never be raised in relation to his own heterosexual contact with non-commercial partners. Since the heterosexual partners of those individuals involved (whether as prostitutes or as clients) in commercial sex are largely unaware of this involvement, few are thus likely to perceive themselves at any special risk of HIV infection, or to take any particular precautions as a response to perceived risks.

In short, then, the specific construction of male prostitution in Brazil opens up the possibility of HIV infection in a variety of different ways for a variety of different individuals, and an examination of the social and cultural particularities of this universe can lead to an understanding of the dynamics of HIV transmission within these populations in ways that would otherwise be impossible. At the same time, however, this understanding of the social universe within which male prostitution takes shape offers important implications for HIV prevention and health promotion. Precisely because it is possible to define the different actors that are in one way or another involved in prostitution, and the distinct territories that serve as their stage, it is also possible to begin to think about the most effective ways to reach these populations, and to develop intervention strategies that respond to their diverse needs.

The ways in which ethnographically informed research on HIV transmission and AIDS might ultimately be linked to more effective interventions and clearer policy decisions are diverse, and should be explored in greater detail than is feasible here. Yet precisely because it is possible to identify groups and territories in relatively specific ways, and to understand the systems of meanings within which male prostitution, bisexual behaviour and the like take shape, it is possible, as well, to draw on these accounts in developing concrete strategies for AIDS prevention. An understanding of sexual geography can be used to identify points of access for groups that have been viewed as hard to reach. The social and cultural classification of different groups (*michês, travestis, mariconas, fregueses, bofes* and so on) interacting within these territories can offer insight into ways of more effectively segmenting populations for education and health promotion activities. The key point is that while more quantitative investigations of risk behaviour may offer insights into some aspects of HIV transmission within these population groups, anthropological and ethnographic investigation can perhaps more effectively tie an understanding of the social and cultural dynamics of HIV transmission to the ultimate goal of HIV prevention (Parker and Carballo, 1990).

Ultimately, by situating sexual conducts such as male prostitution or bisexual behaviour within a wider social and cultural context, and examining not merely frequency of discrete behavioural acts, but the complex systems of meaning that structure or shape such behaviours, ethnographic description and anthropological analysis can thus potentially play a key role in contributing to the social epidemiology of HIV and AIDS. Perhaps even more important, precisely because of their focus on the question of meaning, cultural analyses can begin to build a bridge from social epidemiology to more effective strategies for HIV/AIDS prevention (see Parker, 1992). Focusing on the meaning that risk-related behaviours hold for social actors within specific contexts, ethnographic studies can offer the kinds of insights that will ultimately be necessary if social and behavioural research findings are ever to be translated into meaningful interventions or health promotion activities capable of effectively responding to HIV transmission and AIDS in diverse social and cultural settings.

Notes

1   The data presented in this article have been collected through long-term ethnographic observation carried out in Rio de Janeiro, Brazil, from June to August 1982, from July 1983 to June 1984, from July to August 1985, and from June 1988 to the present. While the focus of the current article is principally on qualitative ethnographic data, additional statistical data have also been collected through a survey of sexual behaviour on the part

of male prostitutes and their sexual partners in Rio de Janeiro, conducted between January and December 1991.

2 For analyses of female prostitution in Brazil, see, for example, Gaspar, 1985; Freitas, 1985.

3 The term '*travesti*' is a general category that can refer to a number of quite distinct forms of gender-crossing in contemporary Brazilian society, and a variety of other categories (such as *transformistas* or 'transformers') is often subsumed by the more general notion of *travestismo* (transvestism). My focus in this essay will not be on the complex distinctions that can be found in the social and cultural construction of transvestism in Brazil (a subject which should be explored more fully in its own right), but on the social construction of one particular type of transvestism linked to the practice of prostitution in major urban centres.

4 For a fuller discussion of the notion of 'sexual geography', and of its potential usefulness for the ethnography of sexual communities and sexual behaviour, see, in particular, Parker and Carballo, 1990.

5 The focus here is primarily on street prostitution. A somewhat different social and economic profile characterizes *michês* working in more closed settings, such as bars, discos and saunas in urban centres such as Rio de Janeiro or São Paulo. Nonetheless, street prostitution tends to be far more common in all major cities, and the profile characterizing *michês* working the streets is thus more pronounced and even stereotypical than the profiles found in these other settings.

6 The reasons for preferring active or passive roles may vary, and can be as much a function of sexual preference as of the complex processes involved in the transformation of the body. The use of hormones, for example, may make erection difficult, and can cause some *travestis* to avoid areas where clients are more likely to want active partners. The link between social class and active or passive preference is complex, although *travesti* informants themselves describe lower-class clients as less likely to take the passive role in interactions with *travestis*.

7 Group living situations are not only cheaper, but also afford the *travestis* a certain degree of protection from both stigma and even violence. To the extent that this provides a social support network that might offer a context of support for risk reduction, it contrasts with the typical living situations of many of the *michês*, whose lives, as has already been pointed out, tend to be far more compartmentalized.

8 It is important to note that preliminary data collected on the incidence of risk behaviours among *michês* and both their commercial and their non-commercial partners suggest that 'business sex' is more likely to be protected than 'recreational sex', as it is perceived to pose risks that are not perceived in non-commercial relations.

Chapter 6

After AIDS: Changes in (Homo)sexual Behaviour

Richard Parker

In Brazil, as elsewhere, the transmission of HIV has taken place above all else through sexual contacts. For a variety of reasons that have already been examined (see, for example, Chapters 1 and 4 in this volume), heterosexual transmission, in particular, has increased rapidly in recent years. At the same time, same-sex relations between men have nonetheless continued to be central to the epidemiology of AIDS in Brazil, accounting for nearly half of the total number of AIDS cases reported in the country as a whole. And although the relative importance of homosexual transmission, *vis-à-vis* heterosexual transmission, has fallen rapidly, the incidence of HIV infection, as well as cases of AIDS, among men who have sex with men in Brazil, have nonetheless continued to climb (Ministério da Saúde, 1992).

In spite of statistics linking HIV infection to sexual behaviour, and to homosexuality and bisexuality in particular, social and behavioural research on sexual conduct in Brazil has been very limited. Until very recently, no substantial surveys of sexual behaviour had been carried out on the population as a whole, and no studies of homosexual and bisexual conduct on the part of males had been conducted. Ethnographic research (such as that described in Chapters 4 and 5 in this volume) had documented the emergence of complex subcultures linked to same-sex practices among males in large urban centres such as Rio de Janeiro and São Paulo (where the vast majority of Brazil's AIDS cases have been reported), but no systematic research had been carried out on the actual behaviours of individuals involved or the ways in which these behaviours have been linked to the spread of HIV. This general lack of knowledge about such an important aspect of the AIDS epidemic, in turn, has limited the ability not only of policy-makers and planners, but also of community-based organizations, to address the complicated issues involved in HIV transmission — and to design effective, socially and culturally appropriate intervention and education programs aimed at slowing the spread of the epidemic.

As a first step toward addressing these issues more effectively, in June 1989 a study of homosexual and bisexual sexual practices and AIDS awareness (AIDS-related knowledge, attitudes and beliefs) among males was initiated in Rio de Janeiro. This project sought to combine both quantitative and qualitative research methods in collecting data not only on the incidence of specific homosexual and bisexual behaviours, but also on the wider social context within which such practices take place and acquire meaning. In an initial phase of rapid assessment and background research, a review of the existing literature on homosexual and bisexual behaviour in Brazil was carried out (see Guimarães *et al.*, 1992), and contextual data on the social and cultural organization of same-sex sexual practices were collected through ethnographic observation and description. Following this rapid assessment, in a second phase of the project 503 structured interviews were conducted with informants from different socio-economic backgrounds. Finally, in a third phase of research, an additional 100 open-ended interviews were carried out in order to collect further in-depth, qualitative data on the meanings associated with different sexual practices as well as with HIV/AIDS and related risk reduction strategies.[1] This chapter offers an overview of preliminary findings from these research activities, documenting the kinds of behavioural changes that seem to be taking place within the population of men who have sex with men in Brazil in the late 1980s and early 1990s, while at the same time pointing to the implications of such findings for more effective AIDS prevention activities in the future.

Changes in (Homo)sexual Behaviour in Brazil

Since the emergence of the AIDS epidemic in the early 1980s, its impact on the gay communities of Western Europe and North America has led to extensive research on homosexuality and bisexuality in these regions. Numerous studies, carried out in major urban centres, have examined the relationship between homosexual or bisexual practices and the spread of HIV/AIDS, and repeated follow-up studies, carried out over a number of years, have made it possible to document both significant behavioural diversity as well as, in some instances, a high degree of behavioural change in response to the AIDS epidemic. This, in turn, has made it possible more effectively to evaluate and design AIDS interventions directed to gay and bisexual men (see Cohen, 1991; Turner *et al.*, 1989).

Studies already carried out in major urban centres such as San Francisco, Amsterdam and Paris have thus opened important ground for the examination of similar issues in other sites. For the most part, however, parallel or comparable projects have not been implemented outside Western Europe, North America and Australia, where a well defined and developed gay community already exists and can serve as the focus for research on homosexual and bisexual practices. While homosexual and bisexual practices exist elsewhere, and may play an important role in the epidemiology of AIDS, significant differences in the social and cultural organization of such practices, their often clandestine nature and a relative lack of a distinct gay community organized around a shared sense of sexual identity have all perhaps combined to limit the development of significant, comparable research on homosexual and bisexual behaviours outside the major urban centres of the fully industrialized West (see Parker and Carballo, 1990).

Within this context Brazil offers an important possibility for the development of research that will be, at one and the same time, roughly comparable with studies already carried out elsewhere, yet also sensitive to the social and cultural specificity of sexual life. Indeed, precisely because extensive ethnographic research has documented the existence of complex (homo)sexual subcultures in Brazilian life, the potential for developing a more complete database on sexual behaviour and behaviour change among the population of men who have sex with men in Brazil is especially significant. Within this context, and in comparison with the somewhat different settings of the gay communities in the United States or the countries of Western Europe, it might be possible to begin to explore the diverse social and cultural factors that influence different responses to HIV/AIDS — and, in particular, the role that cross-cultural differences in social support and community structures may play in the development of risk reducing behavioural change.

Sexual Identity and Sexual Behaviour

These issues emerge with particular clarity when one examines the results of the study carried out among men who have sex with men in late 1989 and early 1990, when more than 500 interviews were carried out with men recruited through social networks and street outreach in metropolitan Rio de Janeiro.[2] The complex relationship between sexual identity and sexual behaviour, already highlighted in ethnographic description, for example, was immediately apparent. A range of different constructions of self clearly characterized the men interviewed; and the very notion of sexual identity was problematic for many. When asked what term they use to describe themselves sexually, fully 24.5 per cent of those involved in the survey failed to respond at all. An additional 8.5 per cent responded using idiosyncratic terms drawn from Brazilian popular culture.

Still, it is worth noting that although only 4.8 per cent of the men interviewed described themselves as 'gay', 50.1 per cent described themselves as 'homosexual' and another 12.1 per cent of the respondents described themselves as 'bisexual' — which might suggest a growing importance for this medical/scientific system of sexual classifications in Brazil (see Chapter 4 in this volume). Indeed, this may underline the extent to which AIDS itself has perhaps played a role in transforming the conceptual landscape of sexuality in Brazil, since it is above all else in relation to AIDS, and the discussion of AIDS-related issues, that the notions of 'homosexuality' and 'bisexuality' have been most widely disseminated in recent years. At the same time it may also indicate that the men participating in the study, and recruited in large part through homosexual friendship networks, are more fully integrated within the gay or homosexual subculture than is true of the more general population of men who have sex with men.[3]

The complicated relationship between such classifications and actual sexual behaviour is especially evident in relation to bisexuality. Of the sixty-one men interviewed who described themselves as 'bisexual', for example, only twenty-four had in fact had sexual relations with female partners during the six months prior to being interviewed. On the other hand, of the eighty-eight (17.5 per cent of the total) men who reported vaginal intercourse with a female partner during the previous six months, only twenty-four (27.3 per cent of the behaviourally bisexual subsample) described themselves as 'bisexual'. The other behaviourally bisexual men described themselves as 'homosexual' (13.6 per cent), 'gay' (2.3 per cent), or some other category (12.5 per cent). Fully 44.3 per cent of the behaviourally bisexual men simply failed to respond, again suggesting the difficulty of classifying behavioural patterns that fail to fit into the neatly ordered categories of medical/ scientific sexuality.

AIDS Awareness and Risk Perception

The fact that AIDS may have played a role in at least partially redefining the categorization and classification of sexual identities in Brazil is itself a sign of the impact that it has already had, especially within the homosexual subculture. This is confirmed by the degree of basic knowledge and information that the men who participated in the survey exhibited in relation to HIV infection and AIDS. While there is significant disagreement concerning exactly when they heard of AIDS for the first time, 98 per cent report having become aware of the epidemic by 1989. The remaining 2 per cent failed to respond apparently because the question was phrased in such a way that they were forced to remember a date rather than simply to confirm being aware of AIDS.

If there is some uncertainty concerning precisely when they first learned of AIDS, however, there is a relatively high degree of agreement concerning many of the most basic facts about HIV/AIDS. Fully 94.2 per cent of the men interviewed confirmed that HIV is definitely or probably transmitted through semen, and 97.8 per cent confirmed that HIV is definitely or probably transmitted through blood. The potential importance of condoms to avoid infection is also relatively well known, with 88.7 per cent confirming that the use of condoms can definitely or probably protect against HIV transmission. There would even seem to be at least some understanding of the distinction between HIV infection and AIDS, with 92.4 per cent believing it to be definitely or probably true that because of the long incubation period before symptoms of AIDS appear HIV can be transmitted by an individual who appears perfectly healthy.

Relatively less certainty seems to be associated with a range of other aspects of HIV/AIDS, however. Only 24.7 per cent of the men interviewed believe that it is definitely false that HIV is transmitted in saliva, for example; and the potential risk that may be associated with both kissing and, in particular, oral sex seems to be unclear. Given the frequent discussion of promiscuity as a key factor in HIV transmission, together with government publicity campaigns focusing on partner reduction as a key to AIDS prevention, it is perhaps not surprising that 81.9 per cent of those interviewed believe it is definitely or probably true that reducing the number of sexual partners reduces one's risk of HIV infection, while 88.3 per cent agree either partially or completely that carefully choosing one's partners is imperative to avoiding HIV. At the same time, however, 79.3 per cent believe that it is definitely (48.3 per cent) or probably (31 per cent) true that it is not the number of partners but the specific things that one does with one's partners that determine level of risk.

A similar degree of ambivalence can be found in relation to anal intercourse, which, in spite of a widespread association with the risk of HIV infection, is nonetheless the focus of significant contradictions in attitudes and beliefs. Indeed, 68.4 per cent of the men agree that anal intercourse poses a life threat; 66.4 per cent state that they would not agree to practise anal intercourse without a condom; and 62.4 per cent agree partially or completely that the use of condoms during anal sex can avoid the risk of HIV transmission. Yet 51.5 per cent also believe that safer sex is difficult in the heat of passion; 48.1 per cent consider anal sex to be much more exciting than safer sex practices such as mutual masturbation; while 51.3 per cent disagree that anal sex with condom use in fact avoids HIV transmission. These contradictions become even more complicated in open-ended, in-depth interviews, as informants confirm the risks associated with anal sex but simultaneously discuss the possibility that a range of additional practices (such as douching or other forms of hygiene) following intercourse may be sufficient to reduce this risk.

Ultimately, then, while a high degree of information seems to be available about the most basic facts of HIV/AIDS, a good deal less clarity is found in relation to more complicated issues (such as the relative risk of oral sex) and more complex subjective questions (such as the erotic meaning of anal intercourse or the negotiation of safer sexual practices). This is in keeping with predominant sources of information about HIV/AIDS currently available in Brazilian society, and the relative lack of community-based support structures that might permit more effective approaches to the complicated and intimate meanings associated with sexual behaviour change, particularly among men who have sex with men. The vast majority of AIDS education and information takes place in relatively simplistic and highly impersonal ways through the mass media: 82.9 per cent of the men interviewed acquire information about AIDS through television, 78.7 per cent through newspapers and 54.1 per cent through radio. More personal, or community-based settings play a much less significant role: although 65.6 per cent report receiving AIDS information through friends and family, only 19.5 per cent mention the context of a clinic or medical centre, only 6.4 per cent mention school, only 2.2 per cent mention church or a religious centre, and only 2.8 per cent mention government officials or authorities.

In particular, it is worth nothing the relatively limited importance of gay community organizations in providing information and support in relation to HIV and AIDS in Brazil, precisely because this contrasts so markedly with the situation in many other societies. While commercial establishments such as bars and saunas seem to play an important role in the lives of many respondents, only 13.3 per cent of the men interviewed report having had the experience of working with local gay organizations or groups; and it would appear that the AIDS prevention activities developed by such organizations, while clearly of great value, have generally not had a significant impact on the lives of the vast majority of men who have sex with men in Brazil.

Self-Reported Behaviour Change

Given this somewhat contradictory profile of general knowledge and information mixed with many specific doubts or contradictions concerning HIV/AIDS, together with a serious lack of community support structures that might reinforce risk reducing behavioural change, it is worth emphasizing that a significant percentage of the men interviewed reported having made behavioural changes in response to the epidemic, although the nature of these changes is not always clear and the degree to which they have been implemented is not always fully consistent. Only 15.1 per cent reported having made no change in their sexual behaviour, while 40 per cent claimed to have made 'many' changes, and an additional 31.8 per cent reported having made at least 'some' changes. In general terms, as in many other studies of homosexual and bisexual behaviour change in relation to HIV/AIDS, these changes seem to be characterized above all else by (1) a relative increase in non-penetrative sexual practices such as solitary and mutual masturbation; (2) a decrease in both active and passive anal intercourse; (3) a slight reduction in oral sex, as well as in orgasm during oral sex; and (4) a general increase in the use of condoms.

In relations with regular partners, for example, 27 per cent of those interviewed report having diminished the frequency of passive anal intercourse, while 26.8 per cent have diminished the frequency of active anal intercourse. An additional 8.2 per cent report having discontinued altogether passive anal intercourse, while 5.4 per cent have stopped engaging in active anal intercourse. At the same time 24.1 per cent reported having begun to use condoms in relations with regular partners, while 12.9 per cent reported having increases the frequency of condom use.

Reduction in rates of passive and active anal intercourse and increases in condom use with regular partners have been accompanied by reductions in oral sex both with and without ejaculation, as well as by an increase in the frequency of mutual masturbation. While 5.2 per cent reported having stopped engaging in oral sex without ejaculation, 14.5 per cent reported having discontinued engaging in oral sex with ejaculation. An additional 22.3 per cent have diminished the frequency of oral sex without ejaculation, while 17.5 per cent have diminished the frequency of oral sex with ejaculation. Finally, 2.8 per cent reported having begun practising mutual masturbation with their regular partners, while 20.7 per cent have increased the frequency of mutual masturbation.

Interestingly, although many studies of homosexual and bisexual behaviour change in response to HIV/AIDS have emphasized significant differences in behavioural change with casual as opposed to regular partners, in the current study of Brazilian men these differences were relatively less significant. The most marked differences were found in relation to anal intercourse, with 15.9 per cent reporting having stopped engaging in passive anal intercourse and 11.3 per cent having discontinued active anal intercourse with casual partners — approximately twice the percentage reporting similar changes in relations with regular partners. An additional 25.8 per cent reported having reduced the frequency of passive anal intercourse with casual partners, while 28.4 per cent reported reducing the frequency of active anal intercourse — roughly comparable to the frequencies reported in relations with regular partners. As in regular partner relations, 25.2 per cent reported having begun to use condoms, and 13.3 per cent reported having increased the frequency of condom use.

Finally, and again similar to the rates reported in regular partner relations, 7.8 per cent of the sample reported having discontinued oral sex without ejaculation, and an additional 24.3 per cent reported having reduced the frequency of this practice with casual partners. Oral sex with ejaculation had been discontinued by 17.9 per cent, while exactly the same percentage had reduced its frequency. Again, almost exactly as in regular partner relations, 2.6 per cent had begun to engage in mutual masturbation with casual partners, while 19.3 per cent had increased the frequency of mutual masturbation. An additional 23.3 per cent reported having increased the frequency of solitary masturbation as a result of the risk of HIV/AIDS.

With the exception of significantly higher rates of reduction in relation to both passive and active anal intercourse with casual partners, then, the incidence of self-reported behavioural change showed relatively little of the significant differentiation between regular and casual partners that seems to have characterized similar studies in other social and cultural settings. Indeed, this fact perhaps highlights the extent to which regular partner relations in Brazil, where homosexual subcultures are clearly evident but little in the way of an organized gay community can be found, may take very different forms than in societies where gay communities and lifestyles are differently structured. Indeed, only 7.2

per cent of the sample reported living with a male sexual partner. While 29.6 per cent reported being involved in a 'closed' relationship and 33.4 per cent in an 'open' relationship, 48.1 per cent reported having a single regular partner and only 14.6 per cent reported having more than one regular partner. Fully 48.7 per cent of the respondents reported having had no casual partners during the month prior to being interviewed, and only 51.3 per cent reported one or more casual partners during the previous month.

In short, it would appear that ongoing regular partner relations between men are relatively common in Brazilian society — as common, in fact, as casual partner relations. There would appear to be relatively less space for the institutionalization of these relationships, particularly through the establishment of common living situations, as may more frequently take place in the gay communities of North America or Western Europe. Parallel or simultaneous regular and casual partner relationships seem to be relatively uncommon — less common, perhaps, than sequential, and often short lived, regular partner relations. Perhaps as a result of this, the subjective response of informants to regular partner relations may not be significantly different than to casual partner relations; and the tendency to downplay safer sexual practices in regular partner relations, while practising safer sex with casual partners, may not be as pronounced as has been found to be the case in studies of sexual behaviour and behaviour change in some other societies.

Self-Reported Risk Behaviour

While a relatively high degree of AIDS awareness, marked by widespread concern about the epidemic and the risks that it poses together with a significant degree of information about HIV transmission, would thus seem to be linked to important behavioural changes among homosexual and bisexual men, data on the continued incidence of risk behaviours suggest that the risk of HIV transmission among men who have sex with men in Brazil continues to be significant. In spite of the important behaviour changes reported by respondents, high risk behaviour continues to be a part of the sexual repertoire, of a significant percentage of the men interviewed. Indeed, it would appear that even many of the individuals reporting behavioural changes continue to practise a range of high risk behaviours — that behavioural change is often inconsistent and partial. By extension, both ethnographic investigation and in-depth open-ended interviews suggest that a general lack of social and community support structures may be associated with a significant degree of psychological or subjective conflict and contradiction concerning sexual excitement, risk perception and consistent adoption of safer sexual practices (see also Costa, 1992).

In spite of reported changes in the practice of oral sex, for example, 78.6 per cent of the men interviewed reported having fellated another man during the six months prior to interview, while 71.2 per cent reported having been fellated. Fully 53.3 per cent had received the ejaculate of their partners, and 52.1 per cent had ejaculated during oral sex. Only 16.9 per cent had performed fellatio with their partner using a condom, and only 12.1 per cent had used a condom while receiving fellatio.

As has already been mentioned, significant doubt continues to exist concerning the relative risk of oral sex with and without ejaculation, and the continued incidence of fellatio even with ejaculation clearly reflects a general sense that it poses less risk than other sexual practices such as anal or vaginal sex. At the same time, however, the erotic value assigned to oral sex, particularly with ejaculation, is clearly important, as 45.7 per cent of the men interviewed consider performing oral sex to be highly exciting when their partner ejaculates. Although 37.4 per cent continue to view fellatio as highly exciting when their partner removes his penis before ejaculating, oral sex with condoms is nonetheless stereotypically described as *'chupando bala com papel'* ('sucking a candy with the wrapper on'). Even more striking, while 74.2 per cent view being fellated as highly exciting when they ejaculate in their partner's mouth, only 48.3 per cent consider it highly exciting when they remove their penis in order to ejaculate.

Although anal sex is correctly perceived as posing a far greater risk of HIV transmission than oral sex, it nonetheless remains nearly as frequent a part of the sexual repertoire of respondents as is oral sex. Fully 67.4 per cent of the men in the survey reported having engaged in active anal intercourse with a male partner during the six months prior to being interviewed, while 65.6 per cent reported receptive anal intercourse. Of the total sample, 55.9 per cent reported having ejaculated while penetrating their partner, while 55.7 per cent reported that their partner ejaculated while penetrating them. Fully 54.1 per cent of the respondents reported having penetrated a partner without a condom during this period, while only 34 per cent reported having done so with a condom, and 47.3 per cent reported having been penetrated without a condom, while only 35.4 per cent reported having been penetrated by a partner using a condom.

As in the case of oral sex, this continued high incidence of anal sex, independent of its perceived risk and apart from self-reported reduction in its frequency, suggests an ongoing inconsistency and a significant degree of psychological conflict in relation to the adoption of safer sexual practices. While 75.3 per cent view penetrating another man and ejaculating in his anus as highly exciting, and 74 per cent think that it is highly exciting to penetrate another male without using a condom, only 29.2 per cent view penetrating a male partner while using a condom as highly exciting. Similarly, while 63.2 per cent view being penetrated by another man who ejaculates in them as highly exciting, and 62 per cent consider it highly exciting to be penetrated by a man who is not using a condom, only 28.6 per cent consider being penetrated by a man who is using a condom to be highly exciting.

These responses are confirmed in in-depth open-ended interviews by informants who suggest that condom use continues to be seen not only as unerotic but as a significant barrier to sexual intimacy. The introduction of condoms into sexual scripts is considered especially difficult — an '*abaixo tesão*' (literally, 'bring down excitement') that profoundly inhibits the development of the sexual act. Further inconsistency, along with the complicated associations linking condom use to the inhibition of sexual and emotional intimacy, can be found as well in repeated cases of condom use early in the development of regular partner relations, but the relatively frequent, and relatively quick (often in less than six months), discontinuation of use as the relationship becomes more profound. After time, abandoning condom use becomes a sign of trust and intimacy within the relationship, in spite of survey respondents' claims to increased condom use even with regular sexual partners.

In short, then, in spite of high levels of self-reported behavioural change, associated at least in principle with a reasonably high degree of knowledge and information about HIV transmission and AIDS, a review of sexual behaviours currently practised by the men interviewed suggests that behavioural change in response to the HIV/AIDS epidemic has in fact been inconsistent and problematic at best. An understanding of transmission and risk reduction seems to contrast sharply with a range of sexual values, deeply rooted not only in the homosexual subculture, but in Brazilian sexual culture more generally, associated with erotic pleasure and sexual satisfaction. This is particularly true in relation to discontinuation of anal intercourse and/or adoption of condom use as fundamental to the reduction of risk in homosexual relations. While further investigation of the subjective meanings associated with such practices is needed to explore fully its implications, it is among the most important findings of the present research, and must urgently be taken into account in the formulation of health promotion and AIDS prevention activities directed to gay and bisexual men in Brazil (see Parker and Carballo, 1991).

Bisexual Behaviour

Since the focus of this study was to gather information on homosexual behaviour and behaviour change, rather than to address the specific question of bisexuality, no concerted attempt specifically to target behaviourally bisexual men was made in recruiting potential inform-ants. Nonetheless, a significant number of subjects (60 per cent of the total sample population) reported having had sexual contact with women at some point in their sexual histories, while a smaller, but nonetheless significant number (17.5 per cent of the total) reported having engaged in sexual intercourse with female partners during the six months prior to being interviewed. This group, defined on the basis of bisexual contacts within a six-month period prior to the interview (and thus offering a relevant time frame for evaluating the relative risk of bisexual behaviour in relation to HIV transmission), can thus be taken as a currently bisexual subsample within the broader sample of men who have sex with men interviewed in this study. Without presuming that this subsample, recruited principally through homosexual networks, is necessarily representative of the broader universe of male bisexual behaviour in the population as a whole, it is nonetheless useful to examine it separately in order to analyze some of the ways in which behavioural differences, within the broader context of sexual meanings and subcultures in Brazil, may be linked to important differences in both risk behaviour and risk reduction.

Perhaps not surprisingly, as has already been mentioned above, of this subsample of eighty-eight currently behaviourally bisexual men, only 27.3 per cent of these men described themselves as 'bisexuals'. While 13.6 per cent of these behaviourally bisexual men described themselves as 'homosexual' and another 2.3 per cent as 'gay', 12.5 per cent described themselves employing some other classificatory category, and fully 44.3 per cent failed to respond at all.

Independent of the ways in which they classify their sexuality, when asked about their knowledge of HIV/AIDS, the majority of the behaviourally bisexual sample showed a relatively high level of AIDS awareness (though less than was reported by the exclusively homosexual respondents). All eighty-eight had heard of AIDS, and 91 per cent reported that HIV is either definitely (75 per cent) or probably (15.9 per cent) transmitted through semen. Though with somewhat less certainty, nearly as many (88.6 per cent) reported that the use of condoms could definitely (50 per cent) or probably (38.6 per cent) reduce the sexual transmission of HIV. Although 22.7 per cent reported having made no changes in their sexual behaviour after having learned of AIDS, another 25 per cent reported having made some changes, and 35.2 per cent reported having made major changes. In comparison, only 13.5 per cent of the exclusively homosexual subsample reported having made no behavioural changes, while 33.3 per cent reported some changes and 41 per cent reported major changes.

As in the analysis of the sample population as a whole, if one examines sexual practices among this behaviourally bisexual subsample, it is again apparent that the incidence of high risk behaviour continues to be significant. High rates of insertive and, to a lesser extent, receptive anal intercourse were reported with male partners, for example, while condom use was reported to be relatively limited. While 75 per cent reported having anally penetrated another man in the previous six months, for example, only 46.6 per cent reported having done so (at least once) with a condom, while 56.8 per cent reported having done so (at least once) without a condom. And while 40.9 per cent reported having been anally penetrated, only 28.4 per cent reported having been penetrated with the use of a condom, while 19.3 per cent reported having been penetrated without the use of a condom.

Perhaps not surprisingly, but certainly no less worrisome, the incidence of risk behaviours with female partners seems to be even more significant. Fully 55.7 per cent reported having engaged in anal intercourse with a female partner during the past six months, and 47.7 per cent reported having ejaculated during anal intercourse with a female partner, while 43.2 per cent reported having done so without the use of a condom. Of the 100 per cent of the sample reporting having engaged in vaginal intercourse during the six months prior to being interviewed, 88.6 per cent reported having done so without the use of a condom. Although 43.2 per cent reported having used a condom in vaginal intercourse during this same period, it is clear that for roughly three-fourths of those men, condom use is at best irregular or inconsistent.

In short, then, within this group of behaviourally bisexual men, risk behaviours continue to be practised with relative frequency, and condom use continues to be relatively limited. Patterns of risky behaviour can be found in relation to both male and female sexual partners, with even more significant levels of risk apparently characterizing heterosexual interactions, particularly due to the lower level of condom use in both anal and vaginal intercourse with women.

The reasons for this continued practice of high risk behaviours are of course multiple, and most probably vary depending on the specific situation in question. Among this particular group, however, data suggest that complicated, and sometimes contradictory attitudes related to risk, sexual excitement and condom use are crucial. Of the men interviewed, for example, 75 per cent classified anal penetration of another male without a condom as high risk behaviour, while only 6.8 per cent considered it risky when using a condom. While 72.7 per cent classified anal penetration as highly exciting without a condom, however, only 23.9 per cent still considered it to be exciting when using a condom. Much the same association seems to hold true in relation to sex with women. Fifty-one per cent of the sample considered vaginal intercourse to be high risk without a condom, while only 5.7 per cent considered it risky with the use of a condom. While 76.1 per cent found vaginal intercourse highly exciting without a condom, however, only 35.2 per cent found it highly exciting when practised with the use of condoms.

These statistics suggest that the perception of risk may not always be enough to overcome a negative image of condom use as erotically unsatisfying, regardless of the sexual practices or partners involved. Beyond this, however, they also suggest that even lower empirical rates of condom use with female partners than with male partners may be linked to a greater perception of risk in homosexual than in heterosexual relations — a possibility that may well be accentuated, in turn, by the fear that condom use (associated in popular thought with AIDS, and hence with homosexuality) may also open up suspicions concerning the possibility of involvement in non-heterosexual behaviour.

Conclusion

It must be emphasized that the data analysis presented here is preliminary. Even in the absence of further analysis, however, it is possible to draw a number of conclusions relevant for confronting the dilemmas involved in developing AIDS prevention activities for men who have sex with men in urban Brazil. While the data show that at least some behavioural change has taken place among the gay and bisexual population in Brazil, it is also clear that this behavioural change has been limited in a variety of ways, and that significant indices of high risk behaviour continue to characterize the lives of many informants. The clearest conclusion emerging from this research, then, is the urgent need for health promotion programs directed to homosexual and bisexual men throughout the country (see also Daniel and Parker, 1991).

This conclusion should be stressed with special emphasis in the Brazilian context, particularly since reports of gay and bisexual behaviour change in other countries have often been interpreted in the Brazilian news media as if they were somehow applicable to the homosexual and bisexual population in Brazil (see Costa, 1992; Daniel and Parker, 1991). At the same time the rapid spread of HIV through heterosexual contacts in Brazil has tended to reinforce the inaccurate perception that HIV/AIDS risks have ceased to be a significant problem within the homosexual population. Clearly, the data collected here do not confirm these popular perceptions. They suggest, on the contrary, that if some behavioural change has taken place among men who have sex with men in Brazil, it has been limited and often highly inconsistent. Condom use, in particular, seems to be partial even among those informants who report that they have adopted the use of condoms in order to protect themselves against HIV infection; and unprotected anal intercourse continues to be frequent.

Equally important, it should be noted that the patterns of inconsistency in continued risk behaviour do not appear to be precisely the same as in much reported research on gay and bisexual behaviour change. There is no clear division, for example, between safer sexual practices with casual partners as opposed to continued high risk behaviour with regular partners. This same contradiction is only minimally apparent in the Brazilian men who were interviewed; and the possible factors that may condition inconsistent adoption of safer sexual practices with different types of partners remain a priority for further study.

Together with inconsistencies in the adoption of safer sexual practices, it would appear that significant emphasis has been placed on the reduction in numbers of sexual partners and the careful selection of partners believed to be uninfected, rather than the adoption of safer sexual practices as an important key to risk reduction. Given the obvious dangers of such strategies, particularly in social/sexual networks that may already be characterized by high levels of seroprevalence, this tendency should be cause for considerable concern.

In addition, as the distinctions between the risk behaviours of homosexual and behaviourally bisexual men make clear, the question of sexual identity, together with an individual's insertion in the homosexual milieu or subculture, may be extremely important in determining different patterns of risk behaviour. Men who are less clearly gay identified, or who are more disconnected from the networks of friendship and solidarity that might offer social support for behavioural change, appear to maintain higher levels of risk behaviour; and complicated ideological structures (such as the problematic association of homosexuality with HIV/AIDS) raise serious psychological conflicts for some men.

These points are aggravated further by the general lack of a developed gay community, with its own institutions and support structures, in the Brazilian context. The limited number of gay organizations that do exist, such as the Atobá group in Rio de Janeiro, have carried out heroic AIDS prevention activities. Their impact is confirmed by the fact that men who have had significant contacts with such organizations (or with AIDS service organizations more generally) engage in considerably less high risk behaviour than informants who have had little or no contact with such organizations. As has already been pointed out, however, the number of gay organizations in Brazil is extremely limited, and their ability to reach out to the full range of individuals involved in same-sex interactions is highly restricted. In spite of the extremely important efforts of such organizations, then, the number of men who have sex with men, but who lack a system of social and psychological support for behavioural change and risk reduction, continues to be significant.

Many of these same factors that limit support for risk reducing behavioural change generally become all the more intense in evaluating the situation of specific subgroups within the broader group of men who have sex with men. It is clear that behaviourally bisexual men, for example, are less likely to be integrated into those community structures that do exist, and, indeed, may not even identify themselves as homosexual or bisexual. They may be considerably less likely to perceive the need for risk reducing behavioural change, particularly in their relations with female partners, and may be unlikely to respond to health promotion or educational interventions directed to gay men. Much the same can be said, with slightly different twists, of other distinct subgroups such as male prostitutes or transvestites. It is thus imperative to emphasize the need for multidimensional health promotion and education programs in Brazil directed to these different populations.

Finally, it is also important to call attention to the need for health promotion activities and intervention programs that move beyond the presentation of basic information and address the more complicated social and psychological issues associated with safer sex. It is clear that a relatively high level of knowledge and information already exists within the sample population. There are significant doubts remaining concerning some of the more complicated issues associated with HIV transmission, but a relatively accurate perception of HIV/AIDS risk already exists. There is considerable ambivalence about the reduction of risk and the adoption of safer sexual practices, however, that would appear to be largely independent of existing levels of knowledge and information.

Given the existing level of information within the population of men who have sex with men, it would seem important to focus on building up a more solid, social and psychological basis for behavioural change. Intervention programs for men who have sex with men should seek to develop social support structures that will be able to provide positive reinforcement for risk reduction. This may mean reinforcing those structures that already exist, such as gay organizations involved in AIDS prevention. But it may also mean creating new structures, such as counselling programs directed to homosexual and bisexual men.

In addition, intervention programs must clearly address the complex meanings associated with sexuality within this population. The current emphasis on partner reduction and partner selection should ideally give way to a more complex focus on sexual practices related to the risk of HIV transmission, and possible mechanisms for reducing this risk. Condom promotion should be given high priority, but will necessarily have to be presented in ways that address the complicated erotic meanings associated with some risk behaviours, together with the limited erotic value associated with condom use. The eroticization of safer sexual practices should be a high priority; and safer sex workshops might be considered as an important way of moving past existing levels of knowledge and information by providing collective contexts in which men can explore the complicated attitudes associated with condom use and behavioural changes in socially reinforcing ways (see Parker, 1992).

These conclusions obviously raise a range of highly complicated issues that cannot be resolved here, but that must ultimately be addressed in order to develop more effective programs and policies aimed at preventing the spread of HIV/AIDS among the population of men who have sex with men. They are intended principally as a point of departure, to suggest some of the possible implications that the current data might offer to AIDS education and health promotion specialists seeking to address the needs of this population in Brazil. More generally, they may offer some sense of the potential usefulness of social and behavioural research findings in seeking to ground more effective AIDS prevention activities in the future.

Notes

1 This survey of sexual behaviour and behaviour change was carried out as part of a comparative study supported by the then Social and Behavioural Research Unit (subsequently the Social and Behavioural Studies and Support Unit) of the World Health Organization's Global Programme on AIDS.

2 While the representativeness of a sample constructed along these lines is problematic, it is nonetheless possible to point to a relatively high degree of social and demographic diversity among the men interviewed. Of the 503 men interviewed, for example, 20.7 per cent were between the ages of 14 and 21, 34.4 per cent were between the ages of 22 and 31, 25.4 per cent were between the ages of 32 and 41, and 19.5 per cent were 42 or older. Similar diversity can be found in the educational level of the sample, a rough indicator of class standing in a society such as Brazil, in which access to education is closely associated with an individual's socio-economic class: 10.3 per cent of the sample had never completed even primary school, 22.5 per cent had primary schooling, 39.8 per cent had completed a secondary education, and 26.1 per cent had completed some form of university or professional degree. Like educational level, place of residence can be taken as a rough indicator of class standing in Brazil generally, and in Rio de Janeiro in particular, with the largely middle-class *Zona Sul* or South Zone of the city being characterized by a relatively higher standard of living than the lower-middle-class *Centro* or Centre, on the one hand, and the lower-middle to working-class neighbourhoods of the *Zona Norte* (North Zone) and the *Zona Oeste* (West Zone), on the other: only 16.7 per cent of the men interviewed currently live in the *Zona Sul*, while 20.3 per cent live in the *Centro*, 51.5 per cent in the *Zona Norte* and 5.4 per cent in the *Zona Oeste*. Finally, while racial classification is especially complex in contemporary Brazilian society, and is typically shaped by subjective meanings that may vary significantly from one informant to another, a relatively high degree of diversity also characterized the racial composition of the sample: 53.3 per cent of the men interviewed classified themselves as *branco* or white, but an additional 23.9 per cent classified themselves as *mulato* (mulatto) and 19.3 per cent as *negro* (black). As in all survey research carried out in Brazil, this self-reported racial categorization was marked by a tendency toward *enbranquecimento* or 'whitening', which is itself a reflection of the social stigma and discrimination associated with skin colour, but which suggests that the sample can be characterized as relatively diverse in terms of racial composition.

3 Given this possibility, it is important to stress the need for more focused studies, drawing on more intensive recruiting efforts, that would make it possible to gather fuller information about more hidden, and not self-identified, parts of the population of men who have sex with men in Brazil.

Chapter 7

The Politics of AIDS Education in Brazil

Richard Parker

Since the earliest cases began to be reported in the early 1980s, AIDS has quickly emerged as one of the most serious public health problems in contemporary Brazilian life. As in other nations, given the lack of a vaccine or a medical cure for HIV infection and AIDS, it quickly became apparent that, at least in the short term, education and health promotion would offer the only effective means of slowing the spread of the epidemic. Perhaps even more than in many other countries, however, not only the inherent complexities of AIDS itself, but also Brazil's immense social and cultural diversity seem to have raised a series of problems for the development of effective educational programs. In this chapter I examine some of these problems, review the ways in which AIDS education activities on a variety of different levels have sought to respond to them, and look at the possible impact that these educational initiatives have had over a number of years. On the basis of this discussion, it might be possible to evaluate the prospects for AIDS education in Brazil in the future, as well as to offer at least some tentative suggestions about possible implications that the Brazilian experience might have for AIDS education in other settings.

The Social Context of AIDS Education in Brazil

Before discussing AIDS education activities, it is worthwhile to situate this discussion within the wider social context within which AIDS education and prevention have taken place in Brazil. What is perhaps most immediately striking is the remarkable diversity of this context. As stated earlier, Brazil is an immense country, with a territory of approximately 8,500,000 square kilometres, and a population of nearly 142 million people. Extensive regional differences cut across the bonds created by a common language, and social and cultural transformations play themselves out as much in space as they do in history. Nominally the largest Catholic nation in the world, Brazil might just as accurately be described in terms of the no less obvious presence of any number of Afro-Brazilian and spiritualist religious traditions. It is perhaps best described, following Roger Bastide, as a 'land of contrasts' in which the divisions of class, race and gender are evident during almost every moment of daily life, while tradition and modernity somehow seem to exist side by side (Bastide, 1978).

These basic contradictions in the character or quality of contemporary Brazilian life have become all the more evident in recent decades, as the country has undergone profound social and political changes. Unprecedented urbanization has transformed what was once an essentially rural society, stretching, and even at times opening fissures in the basic fabric of social life. No less extensive economic transformations, linked to the complicated politics of both dependence and debt, have resulted in a series of deepening economic crises. Perhaps most important, twenty years of authoritarian military rule, followed by a gradual return to democratic government only in the early 1980s, combined to undercut the basic legitimacy of both civil and state institutions, and left a legacy of neglect and mismanagement in the public health and social welfare systems that has severely limited their ability to confront existing health problems, let alone the problems posed by a new, emerging epidemic (see also Chapters 1 and 3 in this volume).

It is within this context that the AIDS epidemic began to take shape in Brazil during the early 1980s, and both the ways in which it has developed as well as the ways in which Brazilian society has responded to it over more than a decade now have been conditioned by this particular set of circumstances. Like Brazilian society itself, AIDS in Brazil has been marked, perhaps above all else, by its complexity and diversity. While the vast majority of the reported cases of AIDS are found in large urban centres such as São Paulo and Rio de Janeiro, for example, cases have been reported from every state and region, and HIV transmission is spreading rapidly throughout the country. Even greater diversity characterizes the specific modes of HIV transmission in Brazil. Whether one looks at sexuality, the exchange of blood and blood products, or the use of injectable drugs, the complexity and diversity that mark Brazilian life more generally can be found in virtually all of the specific contexts in which HIV infection has taken root and spread (see also Chapter 1 in this volume).

Together with the basic social and economic problems faced by virtually all developing nations, the complexities of Brazilian life more generally, and the diverse social and cultural settings within which the HIV/AIDS epidemic has taken shape in particular, have raised a series of problems for AIDS education and health promotion in Brazil. These problems have been accentuated, in Brazil, as in so many other nations, by both pre-existing prejudices related to many of the groups and practices that have been linked to HIV transmission, as well as by fear and misunderstanding in the face of AIDS itself. The result has been a complicated and troubled situation in which some of the basic strategies and tactics developed for AIDS health promotion in other nations have been able to play an important role, while others have had to be developed to respond to the distinct social and cultural realities of contemporary Brazilian life. In the following section I outline some of the most important AIDS education materials and activities developed thus far in Brazil, and suggest some of the different approaches or strategies that have guided planning and policy-making.

AIDS Information and Education Activities

In reviewing the development of AIDS education and health promotion activities in Brazil, it is perhaps best to think of a number of distinct levels, in terms of both sources and types of information. These different levels can be distinguished on the basis of their content and their specificity; and perhaps all involve rather different degrees of self-consciousness or reflection concerning the basic health promotion strategies that have been employed. Without claiming to have exhausted all of the sources of information and health promotion available in Brazilian society, we can focus our attention on three areas that have been most significant in shaping wider views about HIV and AIDS, and that have most clearly offered an interpretation of the significance of these issues in relation to the population of individuals engaged in same-sex sexual behaviours: (1) the mass media; (2) the information and education campaigns mounted at a national level under the direction of the National AIDS Committee and the Ministry of Health; and (3) the health promotion activities developed at state and local levels, largely through the work of non-governmental AIDS service organizations.

The role of the media in responding to AIDS in Brazil has been mixed at best. On the one hand, particularly during the earliest years of the epidemic, coverage of AIDS was extremely limited. Even when the media gradually began to focus increasing attention on AIDS-related issues, the result was often the production of highly distorted images of both the disease and its perceived victims. The early description of the epidemic, in Brazil as elsewhere, as a kind of 'gay plague', for example, added to prejudice and discrimination against both perceived homosexuals, on the one hand, and people with AIDS, on the other (see Chapter 3 in this volume). Even if sometimes sensationalist coverage has continued to mar at least some AIDS-related reporting, however, the broader response of the media in Brazil has generally become increasingly informed and responsible. Numerous articles in major newspapers and national magazines have focused on AIDS-related issues in relatively responsible ways; and public service announcements and special reports carried on major television networks have increasingly brought the discussion of AIDS into the homes of more Brazilians than would have been possible through any other medium. Taken together, the printed media, radio and television have contributed to the creation of what might be described as a background of basic information — a background that has been crucial in shaping both attitudes and practices related to HIV infection and AIDS.

The importance of television as perhaps the single most important medium for the transmission of information in Brazil has also provided a focus for the education activities of the Ministry of Health's National AIDS Program. As the communication medium that most clearly cuts across the major divisions of Brazilian society and unites the country's diverse geographical regions, television has emerged as the natural focus for broadly based AIDS education and information campaigns that have been developed on a national level since 1986. While posters, pamphlets and advertising billboards have all been employed in conjunction with television, the majority of the attention (as well as the financial resources) focused on AIDS health promotion since that time has been given over to a series of nationally broadcast public health announcements, developed for the Ministry of Health by commercial advertising agencies, emphasizing various aspects of the disease (Rodrigues, 1988a).

The earliest materials developed for these national campaigns focused on the presentation of very basic information: how HIV is (and is not) transmitted, the role of sexual relations, drug injection, blood transfusions and the like. As the national campaigns developed, a strategy emerged in which new announcements would be periodically introduced, successively shifting the focus of attention: an advertising campaign focusing on the potential risk involved in multiple sexual partners might be followed, some months later, for example, by a new announcement focusing on drug injection. Later this series of advertisements was superseded by others, more or less successful in terms of public response, but always aimed at raising AIDS awareness more generally.

Perhaps at least in part because different commercial agencies have been involved in planning the advertisements used in these national campaigns, their underlying messages have sometimes seemed contradictory (ranging, for example, from the early slogan, 'Love Doesn't Kill', to the more recent, 'Don't Die from Love'), and have often drawn criticism from non-governmental AIDS service organizations. In some instances, such as in a particularly ill-fated campaign developed in 1991 and focusing on the lack of a cure for HIV/AIDS, such criticisms have been so severe as to undermine the legitimacy of the technical staff responsible for the federal government's AIDS control program. In general, however, the underlying strategy behind such public service announcements has remained more or less consistent. As one way of responding to the social and cultural diversity of the country as a whole, they have sought to present relatively basic information on different risk behaviours for a relatively general audience, while more clearly focused or controversial messages have largely been avoided (see Rodrigues, 1988a).

This is not to say that thought has not been given to a more careful identification of potential target groups. On the contrary, within its working plan for health promotion the National AIDS Program has clearly targeted at least four broad audiences: (1) health professionals; (2) the public at large; (3) groups engaging in high risk behaviours; and (4) adolescents (Rodrigues, 1988a). The third of these audiences, 'groups engaging in high risk behaviours', has been further broken down into 'homosexual and bisexual men, intravenous drug users, and male and female prostitutes' (Rodrigues, 1988a). There has been considerable debate, however, concerning the most appropriate manner to develop materials for these different audiences, and groups as diverse as gay liberation organizations, on the one hand, and conservative sectors of the Catholic Church, on the other, have exerted pressure from a variety of different directions that has conditioned the development of government-sponsored campaigns (Regan, 1987). While central emphasis has been placed on promoting the use of condoms, for example, some voices within the Church have vigorously criticized this emphasis, and during different periods references to condoms were taken out of government-sponsored AIDS announcements in response to pressure politics. Although the National AIDS Committee has worked closely with a wide range of concerned groups in developing its program, and has managed to achieve a degree of cooperation and collaboration, there is no doubt that a complicated set of political forces has limited its freedom of movement in a variety of ways (Regan, 1987; Rodrigues, 1988a).

Many of the same forces that have limited the federal government's freedom in designing and implementing AIDS education programs have had a similar impact on state and local levels as well. When combined with the severe limitations of most state and local budgets, it is hardly surprising that little in the way of AIDS education and health promotion has emerged at state and local levels in most parts of Brazil. In some more well-to-do regions, such as in São Paulo, more available resources have made possible the development of relatively elaborate and innovative AIDS education programs that have drawn heavily on support from local communities. More commonly, however, as in financially hard-pressed Rio de Janeiro, an almost absolute lack of infrastructure and funding has made it difficult, at least until quite recently, for state and local public health officials to mount more than a minimal response. Even here, however, at the local level important developments have begun to take place in recent years, particularly as a result of the formation of a growing number of voluntary associations and AIDS service organizations that have focused on AIDS education in a variety of different community contexts (see Chapters 1 and 3 in this volume).

While it is impossible within the limited space available here to review the activities of all of the non-governmental organizations that have become involved in AIDS education activities in Brazil over the past five to seven years, even a brief discussion of the activities of key groups can offer some sense of the role that non-governmental organizations (NGOs) and AIDS service organizations (ASOs) have begun to assume in AIDS education and health promotion activities in Brazil. Since the mid-1980s, organizations such as GAPA and ABIA have been among the leaders in the development of AIDS education projects (see Chapter 3 in this volume). One of GAPA's earliest activities in São Paulo, for example, was the production of a controversial poster that drew on highly explicit and popular language to encourage safer sexual practices, particularly among men who have sex with men, and similar, highly focused projects have been developed by the different chapters of GAPA initiated in urban centres around the country in the late 1980s and early 1990s.

Like the different chapters of GAPA, from its base in Rio de Janeiro, ABIA has been heavily involved in developing a set of highly focused health promotion materials directed to a variety of groups within Brazilian society, and has supplied these materials to AIDS service organizations throughout the country. Particularly important projects have included educational videos developed for use with groups such as civil construction workers, street children, adolescents and low income women, as well as informational pamphlets developed for sailors, gay-identified men and HIV infected individuals. Less restrained than government officials by concerns about possible backlash from conservative sectors of Brazilian society, the materials developed by ABIA have been among the most direct and explicit available anywhere in Brazil. They have been distributed to groups working in AIDS education throughout the country, and, along with talks and presentations by ABIA's staff members for audiences as diverse as gay liberation groups, the employees of both state and private businesses and a range of private and professional organizations, these activities have constituted perhaps the most wide-reaching and influential AIDS education program developed by any non-governmental organization.

Not surprisingly, this same emphasis on highly focused or targeted health promotion activities has also characterized a range of different groups and organizations that serve more clearly delimited clienteles. Gay organizations such as the Gay Group of Bahia in Salvador and, particularly, Atobá in Rio de Janeiro have worked closely with a range of other AIDS service organizations as well as with government AIDS programs in developing AIDS-related activities. While the number of gay groups in Brazil is quite limited, and their membership does not include many men who may engage in homosexual behaviours without in any way developing a sense of homosexual identity, groups such as Atobá and GGB have played a key role in reaching out to this population, in distributing both educational materials and condoms, and in offering a range of other support services.

Similarly, working within the Institute for Religious Studies (an ecumenical organization focusing on social and human rights issues), a program focusing on the civil rights of prostitutes in Rio de Janeiro has developed a set of AIDS education booklets specifically targeted to female, transvestite and male prostitutes, and is currently involved in training members of these groups to act as health promotion workers in the specific areas where they work (*Jornal do Brasil*; 1989). Associations formed by prostitutes in different parts of the country have shown an increasing interest in AIDS education, as well as in the social and political issues that the question of AIDS has raised for perceived risk groups in Brazilian society. Together with the activities of more general AIDS service organizations such as GAPA and ABIA, the emergence of specifically focused AIDS education activities rooted in local communities has perhaps been the most significant development in the field of AIDS education in Brazil in recent years. To the extent that this trend continues in the future, it offers the possibility of responding to a set of issues and concerns that may well be, for political reasons, beyond the reach of government AIDS programs, but that are clearly among the most urgent problems that must be confronted in responding to AIDS in Brazil.

Ultimately, then, even if their development has been relatively unsystematic, a range of AIDS education and health promotion activities has gradually emerged in Brazil over a number of years. For the most part, these activities have emerged independently, and, thus far at least, there has been relatively little collaboration or cooperation between different programs or organizations. Nevertheless, even if in largely unplanned and uncoordinated ways, general information available in the mass media, somewhat more specific messages developed in broadly based national advertising campaigns, and more focused or targeted information and education activities on the part of local and community groups have contributed to the discussion of AIDS in a variety of contexts. Together, they have thus begun to respond, at least tentatively, to the complexity and diversity of Brazilian life more generally, as well as to the particular contexts within which the AIDS epidemic has had its greatest impact.

The Impact of AIDS Education

It is far easier to review the different AIDS education activities developed in Brazil than it is to evaluate their impact. None of the educational programs described here has yet been systematically investigated through follow-up research; and it is thus impossible to evaluate the relative efficacy of any particular strategy or source. Even in the absence of such data, however, it is nonetheless useful to identify the criteria that must be taken into account in evaluating the impact of educational programs — the issues that they must address and the effects that they should produce. After these criteria have been identified, it might then be possible, even on the basis of very limited data, to offer some preliminary observations on the initial impact of AIDS education in recent years, as well as some tentative suggestions concerning the prospects for AIDS education activities in the future.

Much of the discussion of AIDS education in general has naturally focused on the question of risk reduction in relation to HIV infection, and both the prospects and obstacles facing educational programs, as well as the definition of success and failure, have been analyzed and interpreted along these lines (see, for example, Fineberg, 1988). Clearly, in the educational response to HIV infection and AIDS, this question of risk reduction is central. At the same time, however, it must be linked to a wider set of issues that, within a fuller definition of the AIDS epidemic, must also be addressed. As part of this broader definition, issues linked to what has been described as 'the third epidemic' — the complex social response to both AIDS and people with AIDS — must also be confronted (Mann, 1987; see also Chapter 3 in this volume). Indeed, it is possible that the question of risk reduction itself can be confronted only to the extent that this wider range of social issues is raised in the discussion of AIDS. Both AIDS awareness more generally as well as the specific questions of prejudice and discrimination should be taken, along with risk reduction, as key questions that must be considered in evaluating the impact of AIDS education programs.

On the basis of the very limited data currently available, the results thus far are mixed, offering reason for both guarded optimism and realistic preoccupation. Data collected in 1987 and 1988 by Gallup International as part of an international survey on attitudes and opinions about AIDS, for example, found that Brazil was one of only two countries in which 100 per cent of the individuals surveyed responded that they had heard of AIDS. No less impressive, 79 per cent of the Brazilians surveyed pointed to AIDS as the most urgent health problem facing the country, the highest total in any of the countries surveyed. Although the question itself may be problematic, in responses concerning the perception of distinct 'risk groups', the data seem to indicate a high correlation between information and education activities, on the one hand, and perceptions of risk, on the other. Of those individuals who responded to the survey, 95 per cent indicated that AIDS is likely to become an epidemic among homosexuals, 95 per cent mentioned people who need blood transfusions, and 92 per cent pointed to injecting drug users, while 67 per cent, an unusually high proportion, saw AIDS as a potential epidemic among the general population. In relation to the more important question of risk-related behaviours, 97 per cent pointed to HIV transmission through blood transfusions and needle sharing, 88 per cent mentioned intimate sexual contact with a person of the same sex, and 84 per cent pointed to intimate sexual contact with a person of the opposite sex (Webb, 1988).

In spite of this relatively impressive degree of AIDS awareness on the part of the general population, as well as relatively accurate perceptions of risk, however, only 14 per cent of the individuals who responded to the Gallup International survey in Brazil indicated that they had made any changes in their behaviours as a response to AIDS.

Just as troubling, only 69 per cent, a relatively low percentage, at least in comparison to many of the other countries surveyed, indicated that people with AIDS should be treated with compassion (Webb, 1988). AIDS awareness, at least on the part of the general population, has thus not necessarily translated into risk reducing behavioural change with any degree of frequency. While the nature of the survey's research design makes it impossible to evaluate the specific reasons for this particular configuration, the relatively low expression of concern for people with AIDS may indicate that ingrained prejudices and pre-existing forms of discrimination in Brazilian society have had an important impact in creating an attitudinal climate that continues to inhibit a more positive response to AIDS-related risks. It may well be that addressing questions of prejudice and discrimination will be as crucial as the question of risk itself in seeking to stimulate risk reduction on the part of the general population.

As in a number of other countries, when one turns from the general population to more specific groups within this population, very limited evidence offers some reason for hope that important changes in both attitudes and behaviours may be taking place as a result of AIDS education activities in Brazil. Given the importance that virtually all sources of AIDS information have placed on the use of condoms as a means of reducing risk, it is important to note, for example, that one limited study conducted by a São Paulo newspaper found that condom use had increased from 6 per cent to 27 per cent among young people between the ages of 15 and 25 between December 1985 and February 1987. The same study found that condom use had increased from 17 per cent to 49 per cent among self-identified homosexual and bisexual adult males — the groups that have had perhaps the greatest access to targeted or focused health promotion materials from a number of sources (*Folha de São Paulo*, 1987).

Similar results have been reported in recent studies of gay and bisexual men in Rio de Janeiro, which have examined the relationship between concern, knowledge and information, and personal experience with HIV infection and AIDS with changes in risk behaviour (see Parker *et al.*, 1989; Daniel and Parker, 1991; see also Chapter 6 in this volume). While extremely high levels of knowledge and information have characterized the populations under study, however, rates of behaviour change have been more limited; and even when risk reducing behaviour change such as increased condom use has been reported, it has been highly inconsistent across time (see Chapter 6 in this volume). In addition, the diversity of the target population has been emphasized, and researchers have underlined the difficulty of promoting behavioural change among the population of men who have sex with men but do not identify themselves as homosexual or bisexual (see also Chapter 6 in this volume).

While such studies have been extremely limited, they suggest more focused AIDS health promotion activities can have a powerful impact in stimulating both behavioural and attitudinal change among specific populations with a heightened perception of risk. They would suggest that, just as increasing emphasis should perhaps be given in the future to addressing questions of AIDS-related discrimination and prejudice, greater attention should perhaps be given to smaller-scale, increasingly focused health promotion activities developed for and by specific communities. As in a number of other countries, the model of health promotion taking shape within, and in relation to, specific communities such as the homosexual population or groups involved in prostitution may well provide a useful model that might ultimately be extended to other communities confronting the risks of HIV infection and the problems posed by AIDS.

Finally, it is important to emphasize the urgent need for research aimed at providing fuller data on the current situation and at evaluating more effectively the impact of specific interventions and educational programs. None of the limited studies carried out thus far has been sufficiently linked to any specific health promotion activity to evaluate its impact or to establish causal links. At best, they offer very limited approximations of what may be occurring, and of why it may be taking place, and it is important to stress the urgent need for more carefully formulated research aimed at the evaluation of health promotion interventions and AIDS education programs (see, for example, Turner *et al.*, 1989). Even as we await the kinds of data that will make it possible to come to informed decisions concerning these issues, however, it is possible, on the basis of the discussion developed here, to offer a number of preliminary suggestions concerning the most reasonable approaches in terms of the overview sketched out here. In closing, then, I turn briefly to some of the specific policy implications that emerge from this discussion, and look at the prospects for AIDS education in Brazil.

Lessons from the Past and Prospects for the Future

In looking back at the history of AIDS education in Brazil over nearly a decade now, it is clear that a number of developments have taken place that offer hope for the future. Perhaps most important, there has been widespread agreement at all levels concerning the importance of AIDS education as the key to confronting the epidemic. No less significant, as data from the Gallup International survey seem to indicate, there has emerged an equally widespread conviction on the part of the general public that AIDS is perhaps the most potentially serious health problem currently facing the country; and this conviction opens the door for the commitment to AIDS education that will ultimately be necessary if Brazil is to respond effectively to the epidemic. Finally, a range of AIDS education and health promotion activities has already been implemented, and a significant amount of expertise has been acquired that may provide a foundation for even more sophisticated and effective activities in the future.

As important as these developments are, however, it is important to underline the fact that there is only limited evidence to indicate that they have translated into the kinds of behavioural changes that will ultimately slow the spread of HIV transmission in Brazil. Even among particular groups such as self-identified gay men, evidence for some important changes in behaviour is limited, and certainly cannot be generalized to the wider population of men who have sex with men. In Brazil, as in other countries, it seems clear that information, in and of itself, is not enough to stimulate risk reducing behavioural change, and that a range of other issues will ultimately need to be addressed in developing more sophisticated and effective health promotion programs in the future.

As an extension of this point, it may be that the most basic goals of AIDS education programs cannot all be met through the relatively general educational programs that have been most pronounced thus far in Brazil. The evaluation of education programs in settings where diverse activities have been undertaken over a period of time has suggested, for example, that behavioural change is most effectively stimulated through highly specific or focused health promotion activities, while more generally oriented activities are better suited to the maintenance of changes over time. Once again, the Brazilian case would suggest that while widespread public service announcements can have an important impact in raising a general level of AIDS awareness, they may well have little impact on the reduction of risk related behaviours. Just as information alone is not enough, unfocused educational materials are not adequate, in and of themselves, to bring about risk reducing behavioural change.

These points offer a number of implications for future AIDS education activities, both in Brazil and elsewhere. While focused or targeted materials have been developed by local and non-government organizations, which have generally had more freedom of movement in this area, they have been the most recent, and most limited, of the AIDS activities thus far carried out in Brazil. During much of the past decade the largest portion of available resources has been given over to more widespread and generally oriented media campaigns. While these campaigns have achieved some success in constructing what might be described as a general background of knowledge about HIV and AIDS, and while this background is no doubt crucially important as a foundation for behavioural change in the future, it would appear that it is not enough to bring about such change on its own.

On the basis of these facts, it would seem reasonable to suggest that the prospects for effective AIDS education in the future in Brazil will be greatest to the extent that it is possible to direct resources to more clearly focused health promotion activities, and to draw on the experience and personnel of the growing number of local-level organizations already involved in AIDS health promotion activities. Thus far, only limited collaboration has emerged between the educational activities of the National AIDS Program and the non-governmental organizations involved in AIDS-related activities, and both a fuller partnership and a commitment to providing necessary financial resources should be taken as important goals for the future. The widespread media campaigns that have dominated AIDS education activities in the past will continue to have an important role to play in the future, both in reaching the hard to reach (the individuals and groups that may, for a variety of reasons, not respond effectively to more focused materials), as well as in contributing to the maintenance of behavioural change where it has already taken place. But the key impact of small-scale, local-level activities in more effectively stimulating such change in the first place should be recognized and acknowledged in the development of complex policy initiatives.

Finally, in addition to rethinking the basic educational strategies that should guide AIDS education activities, careful consideration must be given to the range of issues that must be addressed as AIDS education in Brazil evolves in the 1990s. Attention must continue to focus not only on AIDS itself, but on the wider social context within which AIDS takes place and the wider social responses that ultimately shape the climate of risk reducing behavioural change. Just as some settings stimulate and encourage health promoting change, others discourage it; and addressing the issues of injustice, prejudice and discrimination that might ultimately inhibit a positive response to AIDS must become an even higher priority in years to come. In Brazil, as in other countries, AIDS education activities must therefore respond not only to the epidemics of HIV infection and AIDS, but also to the epidemic of fear and prejudice in the face of AIDS. It is only by struggling with these issues in years to come that it will be possible to build on information itself by constructing an environment that is truly capable of nurturing risk reducing behavioural change in the face of HIV and AIDS.

Achieving these goals, of course, will by no means be an easy task. In Brazil, as in other parts of the world, the AIDS epidemic will almost certainly get worse before there is any hope that it will get better. Confronting it, above all else through education and health promotion, will require collaboration and cooperation on a scale that has not yet emerged in relation to any other social issue. It will require a far greater commitment of human and financial resources than has thus far been made available. The dedicated work of a growing number of men and women, from a wide range of professions and disciplines, along with the tentative steps forward that have been taken over recent years, offer hope for the future. The challenge will be to transform hope into the reality.

Part 3

Living with AIDS: A Personal Perspective

Chapter 8

News from Another Life

Herbert Daniel

From one minute to the next, the simple fact of saying 'I'm alive' has become a political act. To affirm myself as a citizen who is perfectly alive is an act of civil disobedience. For this reason, ever since I found out that I had AIDS, I constantly repeat that I am alive and that I am a citizen. I have no deficiency that makes me immune to civil rights, in spite of abundant propaganda to the contrary.

We all get sick. Everyone will die. Yet when a person has AIDS in Brazil, evil and powerful voices may claim that we are 'aidetics' and, for all practical purposes, provisionally dead until the final hour of passing arrives. I, for one, discovered that what I am is not an 'aidetic'. I am still the same person; the only difference is that I have AIDS — an illness like other illnesses and one loaded with taboos and prejudices. As for dying, I haven't died yet. I know that AIDS can kill, but I also know that prejudice and discrimination are much more deadly. May death be easy for me when it comes, but I won't let myself be killed by prejudice. Prejudice kills during life, causing civil death, which is the worst kind. They want to kill people with AIDS, condemning us to a civil death. For that reason, disobediently, I am striving to reaffirm that I am very much alive. My problem, like that of thousands of other people with this disease, is not to ask for easier conditions of death but to demand a better quality of life. When I first became sick with an opportunistic infection typical of AIDS, between the fever and the fright of having recognized in myself the so-called 'disease of the century', I immediately imagined that from that day on my problem would be how to make sense of my death. Things did not happen that way, although I think that I have seen death close up and have discovered that dying is easier than I once supposed. My greatest worry was not how to respond to the question of whether there is life after death. More important is to ask whether there is life, and of what kind, before death. It is only by responding to this question that it will be possible for all of us to face death, or rather, to make sense of the absurdities that are peculiar to the human condition.

The way I received the news that I had AIDS provoked much greater trauma in me than the simple fact of knowing I was ill with such a serious condition. The doctor I had gone to see, in an emergency, informed me that I was ill, gave me a prescription, charged me 40,000 cruzados and dispatched me from his office. All of this in forty seconds! That was the amount of time he gave me to absorb the shock, while he stared at me with the Olympian indifference of a laboratory technician. To him, I was just a disease, and, what is worse, a homosexual disease. I am convinced that it is prejudice which provokes such a degree of inhumanity, in addition to ignorance about the epidemic. There is violence too, generated by prejudice, which makes people believe that the homosexual is being punished for the guilt he bears.

Situations like this have become sadly frequent. It is difficult in such circumstances to act against the hermetic and arrogant power of the medical profession — a power that enjoys complete impunity. Certainly, there are many doctors who do not believe in practising medicine this way; like the doctors I eventually found who, with solidarity and competence, saved my life during that crisis.

After the clinical coldness of my initial treatment, I became terrified by the prospect of falling into the clutches of a medical machine that, because it knew so little about solidarity, was capable of murder. The AIDS that has been 'medicalized' by technocrats of death is the real horror; it has little to do with the illness itself.

This is the AIDS that has been defined — thanks to a narrow and antiquated view of medicine — as 'infectious', 'incurable' and 'fatal'.[1] This has been monotonously reaffirmed, in the last decade, by all official or officious propaganda about the disease. To present AIDS along these lines is perhaps not to lie, but to promote the acceptance of a half-truth — a vast mythology which is the source of the worst stigmas that the disease carries, and of the worst discrimination against the person who has it.

In the first place, AIDS is said to be 'infectious'. The illness is caused by a virus, HIV, which is transmitted sexually or through the blood. The virus is certainly not transmitted by other means. Since the disease is sexually transmissible, a series of fantasies about its 'infectiousness' has grown from the mysteries and fears generated by ignorance about sexuality. People with AIDS bear the same stigmas as already marginalized groups such as male homosexuals and injecting drug users. All of this drives the sick person underground. Besides being affected by a serious disease, having to live it in solitude, clandestinely, is the worst tragedy that can befall a person with AIDS. To struggle against this imposed civil death, the person who becomes ill must break down the barriers of secrecy. I believe that we must all cure ourselves of shame, guilt and fear. People with AIDS must show themselves as they are, talk about their situation, form mutual help groups and participate fully in society. Such groups, destined to combat the death decreed by going underground, will serve not only as a form of therapy for their members. They will be therapeutic for a society that is diseased with a form of discrimination that creates what has been called the 'third AIDS epidemic' — the epidemic of panic and prejudice.

Second, the 'incurability' of AIDS is merely evidence of the bankruptcy of modern medicine. I say this without any intention of diminishing the seriousness of the illness or alleging that there are miracle cures. For the moment, there is no known method of eliminating HIV from the body; but more and more methods for diminishing its effects are being discovered. To insist on the incurability of AIDS is, above all, a strategy to induce fear, and that is the worst possible strategy for providing health information. The most it achieves is to frighten people and drive them away from real information and effective prevention. Publicizing the 'incurability' of AIDS has other consequences as well. It serves the interests of a host of drug and therapy salesmen, and of various charlatans.

The notion of 'incurability', when interminably repeated, often leads the person with HIV/AIDS obsessively to seek improbable cures. He ends up living under a 'therapeutic dictatorship'. Because he wants so much to be cured, he ends up with only enough time to treat himself, yet without the basic knowledge necessary to make the choices his treatment requires. Since I became sick, I have received the most fantastic offers of 'treatment', alleging infallible and miraculous cures. If I were to believe all of them, I would come to the conclusion that nothing is more curable than AIDS. If I tried all of them, I wouldn't have time for anything else; but I need to plan my life, so I am dispensing with instant solutions.

For people with AIDS, the choice of a therapeutic strategy must be made on the basis of reliable information. Given the opportunity, each person will select a treatment that matches his or her former lifestyle, choosing the methods that he or she trusts. Many people in Brazil — and this is our tragedy — will die without receiving any support from the government for their treatment. They will have to find other means to treat themselves. Above all, however, one must not allow oneself to be deluded, for every illusion carries with it a loss of hope; and maintaining hope is fundamental as a form of therapy in itself.

Finally, simply saying that AIDS is 'fatal' condemns us to civil death. Someone who is contaminated or sick must thereby live another life — a life beyond. The claim that AIDS is fatal has been the basic assumption underlying all Brazilian government initiatives thus far. In a sense this is not surprising in a country which does nothing to take care of its own health, and has not yet realized the seriousness of the AIDS epidemic. There is still no adequate national program to control or prevent the epidemic. There is no information, no support for the ill, no medication, no hospitals. Government bureaucrats, casting a greedy eye upon the international funds spent on AIDS, create programs for foreign consumption and want the sick to die, preferably in silence.

Well, I do not intend to keep quiet. And I am sending those bureaucrats news from right here, from life itself. They are the ones who are agonizing, caught in the quagmire of President Sarney's government.[2] I am alive. And like thousands of Brazilians with AIDS, I demand a change in the course of AIDS policy — so that it is based on an understanding of the seriousness of the epidemic, so that it is defined by social solidarity rather than division. Like every Brazilian, I know that we do not deserve what has come crashing down upon us, a disease of hopelessness. I know, on the other hand, what we do deserve — another life. As for me, I have all the time in the world to build it.

Notes

1 These images are popular cultural constructions rather than scientific facts. HIV is often described, for example, as contagious rather than infectious — indeed, in Brazilian Portuguese, the two notions tend to merge, causing considerable confusion in relation to the transmission of HIV. Such imprecise, and sometimes incorrect, images shape the ways in which society responds to the HIV/AIDS epidemic and those affected by it.
2 José Sarney was President of Brazil from 1985 to 1990. Although he was the first civilian leader of the country after twenty years of military rule, his administration was marked by widespread corruption and a profound lack of responsiveness to the demands of civil society. The first National AIDS Program in Brazil was created during the Sarney administration.

Chapter 9

Above All, Life

Herbert Daniel

> I burst
> at times just
> because I am alive . . .
> (Gilberto Gil)

I know that I have AIDS. I know what this means for me. I try not to have any illusions about it. Only I don't know what other people mean when they say that I have 'AIDS'. Most of the time they mean, 'you are going to die' (but who isn't?). Other times, the more prejudiced say, 'you are already dead' (my daily experience refutes that). Sometimes they sum it up by saying, 'you've lost your resistance' (not yet! Not yet . . . I indignantly resist). In the end, what AIDS is this?

The concept of AIDS was constructed in the last decade, in a worldwide political and ideological battle. The source of the problem lies in the medical definition of what is called, incorrectly, the AIDS epidemic. In fact, the epidemic was caused by several retroviruses called HIV (Human Immunodeficiency Virus), which were transmitted either sexually, through the blood, or vertically (from mother to foetus or baby). Meanwhile, world consciousness adopted the acronym AIDS (or SIDA) as a fact based on, and transcending, technical and medical definitions. Many different meanings nebulously criss-crossed in the dance of words that sought to define the new disease — or if not really new, at least new to contemporary minds and certainly a novelty as a worldwide epidemic.

From a medical standpoint the definition of AIDS was pure fiction. The acronym very primitively referred to a set of signs and symptoms (a syndrome, in medical terminology) which resulted from a deficiency in the body's immune system. This immunodeficiency was denominated 'acquired' to distinguish it from similar congenital conditions. However, similar 'acquired' immunodeficiencies were also seen in radiation victims, in patients who had undergone certain types of chemotherapy (in preparation for transplants, for example, to avoid rejection of the transplanted tissue), in certain leukemia cases, etc. The terms which composed the acronym were enormously uncertain. Explanations for the causes of the disease were still few and incomplete.

Even this layperson's analysis of the acronym shows that it derived from the systematization of some early generic observations about the disease. If critically examined, the acronym reveals how little was known about the disease at that time. Lack of knowledge is less than it was ten years ago, but it still exists today. Meanwhile, the acronym has stuck. The problem is to define that to which it refers, considering the complex circumstances surrounding individual or collective infection by HIV.

The expression 'acquired immunodeficiency syndrome' is as pompous as it is vague. Solemn words that try to say too much say nothing in the end. Surely we have here a formidable display of medical rhetoric. We all know how this rhetoric rushes to cover up, with resoundingly erudite words, the gaping hole of its own ignorance. Where doubt and uncertainty exist, arrogant jargon soothes with an expression that tries to stand for truth. A word, fragile veil of uncertainty, becomes a truth in itself, an ether filling the emptiness that totalitarian knowledge so abhors.

Because it did not refer to anything in particular, the word 'AIDS' began to slide over available significants, thereby producing a signifier for social fissures which previously had no exact expression. AIDS became the syndrome of our days.

It is important to remember that at the time of its first discovery the disease was called GRID — Gay Related Immunodeficiency. It was extraordinary that medical jargon should have come up with the expressions 'gay plague' or 'gay cancer', which later became so widespread. Even more notable was the use of the word 'gay' rather than the term 'homosexual', a clear indication of profound changes at the time in the medical view of homosexuality — no doubt as a result of the gay movement's political effects especially in the United States. A new age was blowing in the wind. Medicine no longer saw homosexuality as an illness, but, instead, subtly began to consider it a source of illness: no longer a pathology, it has become a pathogenic condition.

Medical discourse, replete with generalizing definitions that take on the airs of definitive truths, has drawn upon established taboos to generate the idea that AIDS is either a fatality or a fatal mystery. Yet while much about the disease remains unknown, accumulated know-ledge does allow the assertion that at least AIDS is not a mystery. It is a challenge, but there is nothing magical or fantastic about it. In the end AIDS is an illness like other illnesses. But because medical science knows no more about the disease than the classification of the sexuality of those who have it — understanding nothing of homosexualities — this only results in the fuelling of existing prejudices. The infectious-ness of AIDS, signalled by the ambiguity of the word 'acquired', was conceptually linked to taboos of homosexuality, making the disease a scandal, a terror and a fascination. And because medical science cannot admit, on ideological principle, the idea of death, an intrinsic incurability was invented for the disease. Medical incompetence became AIDS' own destiny, as if its incurability was of a sacred nature laden with ulterior motives.

At present public discussion of the disease has focused on three aspects: its infectiousness, its incurability, and its fatality. In fact, these three myths engender the most distorted and distorting views of the epidemic. Along with the viruses identified as causal agents of the epidemic, an ideological virus has spread in a more generalized and unrestrained manner.

Without resorting to the use of metaphor, it can be said that our society is sick with AIDS — sick with panic, disinformation, prejudice and immobility before the real disease. Effective measures against the HIV epidemic must begin with concrete steps to combat the ideo-logical virus. This means the provision of correct information, effective action, the demystification of fear, the removal of prejudice and the permanent exercise of social solidarity.

For the person who has AIDS or is HIV positive, living with the consequences of the mythologies produced by the ideological virus can be tragic, since objectively mystification kills as much as or more than cellular immunodeficiency. Some dramatic consequences of mys-tification include the inability to fight against infection, failure to get treatment, the resort to 'miracle' cures and charlatanism, and increased violence against people with AIDS and HIV. Two other consequences are the solitude and secrecy with which people with AIDS often feel forced to survive. At the root of the mystifications about AIDS is a series of half-truths based on apparently 'objective' facts, resulting from 'scientific' observations. The 'fact' that the disease is infectious, incurable and fatal has become, thanks to simplification, part of the minimum operational definition society uses to deal symbolically with the disease. Profound prejudices directed against already marginalized groups (principally male homosexuals) re-emerge and are reinforced. Worst of all, the person with AIDS or HIV is declared dead while still alive. Before his or her biological death, he or she suffers civil death, which is the worst form of ostracism that a human being is forced to bear.

There are other problems with the definition of AIDS which reveal the operation of distinctive types of prejudice. The disease's original definition stemmed from North American and European epidemiological research. The fundamental 'model' of the epidemic derived from first world experience, and third world models were the 'exceptions to the rule'. The 'African model' (where transmission is basically heterosexual) thereby serves as a contrast rather than a starting point for understanding the global dimensions of the pandemic. The racism of this ethnocentric view has had devastating effect.

In Brazil, where studies about the disease are still insufficient, Ministry of Health bureaucrats have been fascinated by these 'chic models'. All too often they tried to demonstrate that a 'North American pattern' would apply in Brazil. This has two consequences: (1) to disseminate the idea that HIV/AIDS is an elite disease, coming to our privileged classes from the 'developed world' (an idea which those who work with the disease have proven untrue); (2) to camouflage characteristics of the disease that are unique to Brazil, such as the question of transmission through contaminated blood transfusion (blood continues to be a scandalous issue in our country — genocide is being committed against people with haemophilia and others who need blood transfusion).

In Brazil the disease will affect predominantly poor people because the majority of the population is poor, and any epidemic affects real people in a real country. AIDS is not a foreign disease. The virus is here among us; it is 'ours'. It does not distinguish on the basis of sexual orientation, gender, race, colour, creed, class or nationality.

The epidemic will develop among us according to our specific cultural characteristics — our sexual culture, our material and symbolic resources for dealing with health and disease, and our prejudices and capacity to exercise solidarity. AIDS inscribes itself upon each culture in a different way. Each culture constructs its own particular kind of AIDS — as well as its own answers to the disease. Today these answers depend largely on civil society's capacity to mobilize itself against AIDS and to force the Brazilian government to accept its responsibilities. The current government is still not aware of the epidemic's importance. This government is only a death rattle, ridiculous in its mediocrity, of the authoritarian system which predated it. There is little that looks like a national program to control and prevent the HIV epidemic. As a result, AIDS in Brazil will bear the scars of the government's incompetence.

I know I have AIDS. I know what it means for me to have AIDS in this country. I don't have any illusions about it, even though I am a person with privileges. I am watching many people die as a result of government negligence; I too am dying because of it. We will all die because of it. I know very well what so many living dead mean. I know that I want to shout with them: 'We are alive.' In the end, what AIDS is this which has diseased this (which?) country?

They foretold my death, naming it with an acronym whose four letters do not spell the word 'love'. They are the letters which spell the word 'days' (*dias* in Portuguese), days that we live, or that we survive. I do not want the latter kind of days; I will not accept a predetermined death. AIDS is no more than an illness of our time, like any other, and I cannot agree to their making it a synonym for the final day. AIDS is no more than a viral infection that caused an epidemic which we will defeat, with all the letters that spell love and solidarity.

The days hurt, the last one kills, cautions an old proverb. Thus I am not a survivor. An AIDS sufferer tends to be referred to as a terminal patient with a short survival period. I'm as terminal as a bus station, full of hopeful arrivals and departures to the most incredible and exciting roads that lead to the living. I don't have a survival period; I have a surplus of life, the only one which I can use to leave the trace of a passion that always moved something immobile in me, rooted in a place which I used to call my breast, but which I know reaches beyond any heart. The body, in the end, is disorganized — and AIDS is just an affliction of the organs. Desires are organic disorders. It won't be AIDS that makes me lose my appetite. AIDS only places me, like an explosion of a corporeal truth, in a state of impermanence — something I always lived, but never felt. Let all my days hurt, all of them to the last, as they say of a finger striking the strings of a guitar during a dance.

There, where a truth explodes, passion commands. I am certain that most people with AIDS begin to live passionately from the moment they learn they are ill. Many people naively believe that this passion comes with the explosion of death's truth. As if all that was left for the sick person was the last cigarette before the guillotine falls or before the mercy shot is fired. Death is not a truth. Death is nothing. The truth which explodes in this curious discovery of our mortality — a futile and obvious discovery, although the obvious has become obscure in this alienated world — the truth which bursts forth is the significance of life — before death.

The World Health Organization created one of the first logos for an AIDS campaign, depicting two romantic interlocking red hearts with an unfortunate skull and crossbones drawn between them. The artist attempted to summarize the two earliest and best known clichés about AIDS, associating — as the modern world has come to do — sex with death. Yet, instead of producing an image to describe the new social phenomenon, the HIV-caused epidemic, he created a symbol of prejudice of the utmost gravity: the infectiousness of loving contact, the incurability and fatality of the disease.

This minimal and operational definition of AIDS was the favourite phantom of the 1980s and will probably haunt us for many years to come. The broad social impact of this oversimplification must be countered with efforts directed towards AIDS education and the provision of information, using the voices of those who are HIV seropositive or who have AIDS. Their vital experience contradicts resoundingly the 'minimum definition' and challenges both old prejudices and new forms of discrimination.

This is why I am talking about my illness — in an attempt to demystify a terrible disease that is a threat to the world's public health. It is also my contribution to the effort to disseminate correct information about the disease.

The disease surreptitiously created a mythology so complex that people who have it are seen as special beings, called 'aidetics', in Brazil. Consequently, many people have told me that I have accepted or 'assumed' my AIDS. I find it funny, this business of 'assuming' — an act of will which implies admitting that something exists. What I have done is to assume my place at the door of the world, in order to say: I'm alive; all this talk about my death is an outright lie. People with AIDS must come forward to destroy the misunderstandings created by a corrosive ideology of condemnation followed by pity which has created a melodrama wherein a tragedy is taking place. Undeniably, AIDS is a modern tragedy. It has quickly dismantled the medical and moral assumptions of bourgeois rationality. It reminds us all that pain, suffering and death — as well as pleasure — are integral parts of the world and that no pleasure survives far from the shadow of pain. The world of melodrama, which extinguishes the conflict of tragedy to impose a false egalitarianism in the face of death, can only offer counsel, consolation or consumption: the counsel of a pacification-by-passivity before death; the consolation of forgiveness, only possible if the sinner admits his guilt; and the consumption of soothing therapies that render fat profits to laboratories and other charlatans. The dead — above all, those who have suffered civil death — may no longer be productive, but they are not entirely unprofitable.

For years I lived undercover in Brazil, while fighting against the dictatorship. At the time I kept my sexuality a secret. They were hard times then. Because I fought for freedom, I was persecuted by the police force. During the fight I thought that being a guerilla was incompatible with being homosexual. Later I learned that one cannot fight for half-baked liberties, and that there is no freedom without sexual freedom. Many years ago I came to understand that living my sexuality openly meant demanding citizenship for everyone, not just those who are, or are said to be, homosexual.

To this day, even in large cities and in the most liberal circles, homosexuality is lived either in complete or partial secrecy. AIDS has revealed the most tragic aspect of this living in the shadows. For many, the worst thing is not the disease; it is having to reveal that one is gay, since the person with AIDS is forced to reveal how he was infected. The diagnosis is transformed into a denunciation, so much so that people who do not get AIDS through sexual contact feel compelled repeatedly and permanently to 'differentiate' themselves, so as not to be confused with those who have the very same illness!

I know many people with AIDS. Homosexual or not, their greatest suffering comes from prejudice. It comes from not being allowed just to be sick, but having instead to bear the stigmata of being an 'aidetic'. It means feeling fear due to frequent, yet invisible, social pressures (the worst prejudices are not always necessarily direct discrimination). It means panic at the thought that their sexual and emotional lives may be over. It means the constant presence of those who seem to be waiting to carry your coffin. It means the invisible web of oppression created by family members, sometimes doctors, priests and even friends.

In the face of all this, the most frequent choice is to go undercover — a way of fleeing in order to die, since death is the only kind of life that society seems to offer the sick person. The issue here is not finding better conditions for the sick to die in peace, but finding better conditions for living. Concealment is proof of society's inability to live with this particular disease. It is a testimony to its bankruptcy.

Many people live with AIDS secretly in Brazil, from those who die without knowing they have the disease to those who are killed by discrimination. Sick people who remain anonymous are not able to resist the forces that seek to strip our citizenship from us.

To satisfy this spoliation, tinged by the morbidity of a distorted curiosity, people with AIDS are shown in the shadows, their faces darkened, principally on TV. This is not a way to preserve the sick person's privacy — which is an essential right. It is instead a way of depicting a depersonalized destiny, of fumbling in a region where we all live, unknowingly — it is a darkness that tests our civil rights.

The person with AIDS has become someone without a name or a history. We must take him out of the darkness of concealment so that he can say, in the light of day: 'This is my name, this is my story.' Much more than 'assuming' a 'state of being' or a 'condition', this action will be a collective way for us to write, more democratically, our history.

Nothing has changed in its impermanence: *sic transit*. The experience of finiteness is one of many which weigh upon all mortals. Knowing oneself to be finite is not exactly a novelty. Accepting the body's mortality is more difficult. This is a lesson that the illness brings, and no belief in the immortality of the soul can console the clay which has just discovered its destiny of dust. Certainly, the disease leads us to discover something fragilely different, with a certainty that is anchored in our most intimate depths: life continues. That is, life continues now. There is no death before death — despite the fact that they may already be preparing our funeral, despite the condemnations repeated in the official propaganda. Much remains to be said about this death before death called AIDS, according to the most prejudiced and discriminatory definitions. To speak about it is to shout, 'Long live life!'

I have spoken unceasingly of life — with unfounded optimism. In the end my well founded pessimism says that life is no good and never has been. It is difficult to imagine a day without atomic terror, without class exploitation, without the assassination of forests, rivers and people, without fear, without guilt, without shame — a day which is, shamelessly, just life. Yet there is no other way to find pleasure; we must not only tolerate life but sustain it. And make life a tingle, a jingle and a song. More metaphors! But life is also a poor metaphor — a metaphor for survival in spite of everything. Still, I have always believed, even when I doubted it, that life is the invention of life, the pure creation of the world of humans: to live is not only to transform the world; it is to make it become more beautiful. We have not been too fortunate in this venture. But I do think that one day we will succeed — who knows? One day, one day . . . I mean to say another day. A new one.

People come through and stay a little while. They leave ashes and footsteps behind, which are not always so memorable. It would be better to leave behind only what we would have liked to have done to ourselves. Yet we are what we have done with ourselves. We are what we are made of, this material of time. We are of this time. And many revolutions can mature in this flesh of ours that passes.

My time, my substance, this thing that we have been, myself and I, has not been what I wanted to call 'life'. But it so tempts me that it happens like a precocious pleasure, inevitably — something infectious, mortal and very dangerous inside me. Called 'life', it beats like a challenge. To change, to remodel — one of those verbs or its synonyms — has always stirred inside me, a ravenous thing that has eaten at me from within. This was hope. Hope. This that I always had, in the plural: selves, ourselves, agents of the chaos of light.

Chapter 10

From the Paralysis of Fear to the Response of Solidarity

Herbert Daniel

I am here to tell you: 'I have AIDS and I am alive.' I know that this is a statement about life (and against fear, indifference and horror) that everyone living with AIDS today would like to make to his or her contemporaries. I restate that I am alive to confirm, along with these others, my belief in solidarity.

Two and a half years ago, when I became aware that I had AIDS, being here today seemed implausible to me, since, at that moment, on the best available evidence, I thought my days were numbered. To number one's days is a sad activity. I have learned since that days should not be numbered; they should be lived to the utmost. I have learned that life is the most permanent activity of living. This is called hope, this infectious presence that should occupy our present, as the only assurance of making a better world for everyone. So I gather in my days, as one sows hope, the material of great initiatives that build this immense dream called humanity.

'I have AIDS and I am alive': this statement may seem paradoxical, considering the prejudices that make the person with AIDS a member of the living dead. It is, however, a commonplace fact. After all, life is the only *common place* from where dialogue arises — and love. I am alive, talking to the living, about life. This is my contribution to face the present challenge for this planet, in the end of this millennium: a radical action to defend life.

The necessary and urgent struggle against the AIDS epidemic is part of a great movement to defend life — and to invent life, for to live is not only to survive biologically. It is, as the essence of freedom itself, the pertinency of things and beings to the world: it is the total exercise of one's (so-called human) rights, without which there is only one death, worse than the biological death — a civil death, the absence of every fundamental civil right.

AIDS, in the first decade of its history, brought the seal of exclusion to those infected by the virus. The worst prejudice that surrounded people with AIDS was the one which associated AIDS directly with death. The person infected with HIV became a new kind of pariah, condemned to civil death. A climate of fright was generated: the disease became the 'worst thing' that could happen to anyone, an irredeemable personal and social flaw. This catastrophic view worked to justify, in many cases, immobility in the face of the epidemic, an attitude which preached that 'nothing else can be done.' According to this perspective, AIDS was not only an incurable disease; it was an untreatable disease. The pessimism of these terrorist views proclaimed the defeat of humanity in the face of the virus. But HIV infection is not a synonym for death; the diseases that arise out of this infection are treatable; and, above all, this is an epidemic that can be avoided. Humanity will not be defeated. It will overcome every horror, every prejudice and every discrimination. Life is larger than pettiness and fear. Life is as vast as the love that can unite all human beings.

Yes, I have AIDS and I am alive. I would like to repeat this. Not to convince myself that I am alive. Life is too strong and needs no argument. I insist on this because, with AIDS, I have discovered not only my mortality, but also how great is life's fragility. I have learned that to be alive is to share. To be alive is to be a citizen of my time. AIDS, like any other disease or any other prejudice, cannot reduce one's citizenship. To face AIDS is to face the obstacles to the complete exercise of citizenship. I soon learned that the virus could kill me, but I could not let prejudices destroy me during my life. This is a lesson that must be understood by everyone and every country today. Yes, there is something to fear: the paralysis brought on by fear; the civil death incited by fright. There is something to cultivate too: the dimensions of freedom, extremely rare flowers in these days when gardens are so few.

Living with AIDS is not easy, especially in a country such as Brazil. Living with AIDS in the third world has not been easy. As a matter of fact, living in the third world has never been easy. AIDS has hit Brazil hard. Unfortunately, the government authorities did not provide an adequate response to the epidemic. There have been no consistent information, prevention, assistance or treatment programs. There is not even a proper system of testing and control of blood destined for transfusion. People are being infected by HIV due to a lack of information, to ignorance and disregard. People with AIDS are dying at the very doors of hospitals due to a lack of beds, medicines and health professionals. Public hospitals are in a state of complete abandon, and only a privileged few can count on access to modern drugs and treatments. Nothing has been done to combat prejudice. No concrete measure has been taken against the discrimination that painfully segregates people with AIDS. At the same time, the few government campaigns that should inform the public limit themselves to repeating that AIDS is an incurable, inevitably fatal disease. Indeed, sometimes the government campaigns seem more directed against those who are sick than against the sickness or the epidemic.

This unfortunate picture cannot be attributed simply to lack of resources. In the final analysis Brazil is not a poor country. It is a rich country, with an immense majority of poor people, who are the victims of one of the most unjust systems of income distribution in the world. The inefficiency of the response to AIDS can be attributed to the lack of respect for human rights that characterizes our government. Brazil has been a sad example of how the neglect of civil rights can make the AIDS epidemic grow to the point at which it becomes uncontrollable.

The great challenge of the AIDS epidemic is the struggle to defend basic human rights. Unfortunately, when medical technology is still taking the first steps against the epidemic, many people will die because of AIDS, and many people will suffer the excruciating consequences of infection. Certainly, the poor of the planet will suffer from the impact of the disease. AIDS requires broad measures, or else it will widen the gap between wealthy and poor nations.

The nature of the challenge should be made clear. If, from the medical point of view, AIDS is a disease like any other, against which medicines and vaccines will be developed, we must remember that the epidemic produced by HIV, because of its occurrence in the modern world, possesses complex dimensions that make it far more than a health crisis. They render it a crisis of society, of civilization. In fighting AIDS, we are not only trying to control a biological virus; we are confronting perverse ideological viruses that create a series of social reactions, including panic, ignorance, prejudice, violence and segregation. The consequences of these social reactions can be as disastrous as the HIV epidemic itself.

Against the prejudices that lead to compliance and cowardice, there is one possible response: the response of solidarity. Solidarity is not a vague feeling of sympathy for those affected by the disease. I am talking here about concrete action that values the lives of all of us. Solidarity is a method, a vaccine against the AIDS epidemic.

Today, as we are fighting AIDS, our victory depends upon an

effort not only to defend the rights of infected people, but also to invent a new set of rights for all humankind — rights to understand, rights to prevent, rights to overcome — the rights that turn life into a permanent risk of being solely the right to love.

'I have AIDS and I am alive.' I discovered this when I fell ill. I knew then that one of the first reactions to the disease is to ask: 'Why me?' I soon learned that this was not to be the question. Instead, it should be: 'Why us?' For it does not happen to *me*; it happens to *us*. It happens to humankind today. Being with AIDS links me to all my brothers and sisters, to my contemporaries. The answer to the question lies in the eternal practice of solidarity. Because of this solidarity that turns us into human beings, I can restate, without regret: 'We have AIDS, and we are alive.' We all live with AIDS. Let us make life on our planet an inventory of countless beauties. Let us make a cry of hope sound eternally all over the earth. Let us together cry out, 'LONG LIVE LIFE.'

Chapter 11

You'll Never Forget Your First AZT[1]

Herbert Daniel

Temp, contretemps
cancel each other out
but the dream of living continues. (Drummond de Andrade)

When my doctor, faced with my test results in which figures and ratios indicated that the rules of the biological games played by OKT4 and OKT8 had been broken, pronounced for the first time (and very carefully) the letters AZT as a prescription for my case, I reacted with depression. At first I resisted. After all, I was so well, feeling so secure since I had overcome the first infections. . . . I was not willing to go through the rite of passage that the beginning of the AZT phase represents (or represented to me). . . .

Before the first oblong pill, dressed in its dark blue strip, I made a toast. I was alone in the kitchen, and I said to myself: this is the beginning of the end. And I thought, in my arena, a fatalist gladiator, *morituri salutant*. . . . And, what do you know, everything happened as if I had taken a pill, a pill of any medicinal drug. Nothing creaked, the celestial orbits did not inflect, the floor kept its indifferent rigidity. For some days I kept on taking the drug as if I had been absorbing the Grail that Our Father had compassionately tried to keep from me. Then I realized that I was not taking AZT. I was swallowing, pill after pill, the disturbed metaphors of the medicine; I was swallowing a unique ideology crystallized in the abbreviation and in the news that had been announced about it, rather than in the chemical formula that, a priori, should be restricting the devastating action of HIV on my cells.

AZT, regardless of its chemical composition, has become, in the last few years, part of the complex construction of the mythology of AIDS. Tortuous baroque cathedrals, solid fantasies with domes,

149

needles, atriums, gargoyles and cemeteries were created based upon the virus' biological field of action on the immunological system, and on the difficulties of the relationship between science and a new and alarming disease. Today AZT comprises a seminal element in this delirious process of development; it is one of the essential parts of the ideological jigsaw puzzle called AIDS.

I would like to state that I am not defending AZT. It does not deserve it. It is a drug, and, like all drugs, it has an experimental character; it is not a panacea, and its effects depend on the way it is used and on the person who uses it. I am not trying to construct a pharmacological-chemical argument. The only thing that I want to do, as a layman, is to shake up the laboratory propaganda, the absurd publicity. Advertising drugs, any drug, shows a lack of ethical respect. One should never advertise cigarettes or urodonal, aspirin or Doctor Ross's pills, agrotoxic products or drugs for losing weight. AZT, *noblesse oblige*, gained absurd attention from the media, and, many times, this was instigated by its wealthy manufacturers.

The effect of this action can be evaluated if we simply ask the majority of people the name of a drug used for tuberculosis or the name of a drug used for any problem of the digestive system. Almost nobody knows. However, everybody knows that AZT is used for AIDS. More than that, what seems (but is not) paradoxical, is that the drug helps but does not cure!

AZT became a symbol of one of the foundations of AIDS ideology. One knows that 'aids' — I write the word in lower case to call attention to the signifier that means much more than the disease known by the abbreviation, AIDS — has a minimal operational definition which consists of stating that it is an incurable and inevitably fatal disease. The incurability of AIDS is not a transitory feature resulting from a certain technological stage of medical science. The incurability of AIDS became a metaphysical component of the pathology. AZT comes into play as a soothing drug for the incurability, as a kind of 'mercy shot'. Therefore, the drug is not considered as therapy, but as a tentative (initially frustrated) preparation to an easier death. AZT creates, at least for AIDS, the category of 'terminal disease'.

Based on this ideology, AZT becomes an arrogant instrument, a 'necessary evil'. It is not just a limited, almost humble presentation: 'in fact, this is all we can do for the moment. . . .' On the contrary, it takes the form of an authoritarian imposition that submits the patient to the vision of his mortality: 'bear all the side effects, suffering is always better than dying. . . .' In fact, beneath the piteous rhetoric of a 'minor' or 'necessary' evil is a mechanism for the medicalization of bodies, whose central objective is to capture the patient within a net of powers that have created a true dictatorship of the therapeutic.

The only response to such a trap is the patient's active response, so that he can say to AZT: get back in your place as one of the various possible antiretroviral medications currently available. AZT is a drug with multiple effects, variable reactions, showing excellent results in some cases and not so good in others. But the best result, for each individual, depends upon the user's ability to convince himself that he is simply taking a drug, not a potion full of frightening phantoms and witches from the dark.

Above all, it is necessary to be convinced that while AIDS is still incurable (in the sense that HIV cannot be eliminated from the body), it is increasingly a treatable disease. There are different treatments for every opportunistic disease — and the sooner they are cured, the better the patient's quality of life. More than this, better preventive medications are constantly being developed to slow the advance of immuno-deficiency.

AZT is one of the experiments of retroviral medication. It should be used under control. By saying this, I mean to highlight the doctor's role, but I also mean to draw attention to the patient's own involvement. In this case patience works as a solid instrument for the development of a kind of consciousness that keeps us from being misled by the ideologies of civil death.

I would like to remind doctors that, when prescribing AZT, they should try to cut down the metaphysical forest that it involves for each patient. Explain it patiently. A drug is a drug. Its trips can be good, or have no way back. Information is the key to seeing the possibilities of our own liberation.

For those like me, who have lived the experience of our first AZT, once more I make a plea that we not let ourselves be cheated by therapeutical dictatorships. More than this, we should be aware that, in the case of AIDS, there are several possible therapies, alternative or not, that we should look for. We should act patiently, fully aware of our rights as human beings. We should act with rigour, to avoid being misled by any kind of charlatanism. I have learned that life is full of mystery, but easily drowns in superstition.

Note

1   I would like publicly to thank Walter Almeida, Rosamelia Cunha and Marcia Rachid, who taught me that we do not take AZT with illusions. It should be taken with solidarity and consciousness.

Chapter 12

The Soul of a Citizen[1]

Herbert Daniel

> But anyone who is alive in the world of the living has some hope; a live dog is better off than a dead lion. Yes, the living know they are going to die, but the dead know nothing. They have no further reward, they are completely forgotten. (Ecclesiastes 9: 4–5)

I do not know for how long I have been infected by HIV. I know I was diagnosed in January 1989, when I experienced a series of characteristic infections. From that moment on. . . .

Of course I fear death — not any kind of death, but a special kind of death. However, I have learned not to fear life. I have learned a lot about life, although I know nothing about death, except that I need to learn how to live with it. After discovering that I had HIV, life became a cultivation of living things within myself. I cultivated an inner citizen, a citizen with an open heart. I invented my own soul.

Therefore, I believe I have a lot to say. Not to explain professionally what the disease or the epidemic is about, but to tell what is the challenge of our time: living with AIDS. While I will not be able to describe battles, I hope I can show how difficult the search for balance is. If I consider the statistics, I have been affected by AIDS for a long time. I do not know how long I have been living with AIDS. Maybe decades. However, the most important thing I have realized is that *I am alive!* I have felt well with my AIDS, and I have suffered. It is just a disease after all. I hope that one day, when death finally comes, by chance or by an infection caused by the virus, nobody says that I was defeated by AIDS. I have succeeded in living with AIDS. AIDS has not defeated me. I am a live dog. I bark and I bite. I am winning. I want more people with me, biting . . . life . . . a rare fruit.

The so-called AIDS epidemic — not by itself, but by everything that has been told and created about it — aimed to turn love into a political manoeuvre and death into an obscene metrics. It aimed to transform our heart into a bodily organ, and to stage citizenship as a mortal spirit upon whom it is possible to lower the curtains that isolate the stage of the tragedy as if it were a neutral place in which nothing happens.

The only possible eternity is the interchange of light between each of the human actors who comes on stage: this act of transmission is what we call *solidarity*! The rest is only a superstitious discourse concerning the greed of the infinite. Our scintillation as human beings is our soul as citizens, made with fingers which do not superimpose but entwine; our hands are the mirrors of someone else's hands; our passage through time is the heart that regulates small and fundamental things — since the planet, our planet, which has the exact dimensions of our humanity, beats like a heart.

Life does not win. It happens. LONG LIVE LIFE! VIVA A VIDA!

Herbert Daniel died in March 1992.

Note

1   This chapter was originally prepared for the Eighth International Conference on AIDS in Amsterdam as a declaration of hope and life. It was presented during the closing ceremony of the conference by Claudio Mesquita.

Bibliography

ABIA (1988a) 'AIDS no Brasil: Incidência e Evidência', *Comunicações do ISER*, 7, 4–8.

ABIA (1988b) 'The Face of AIDS in Brazil', paper presented at the Fourth International Conference on AIDS, Stockholm.

ABIA (1989) 'O Número dos Casos e o Caso dos Números', *Boletim ABIA*, 4.

ALEXANDER, P. (1987) 'Prostitutes Are Being Scapegoated for Heterosexual AIDS', in F. DELACOSTE and P. ALEXANDER (eds), *Sex Work: Writings by Women in the Sex Industry*, Pittsburgh, Pa., The Cleis Press.

ALTMAN, D. (1980) 'Down Rio Way', *Christopher Street*, 4, 22–27.

BASTIDE, R. (1978) *Brasil, Terra de Contrastes*, Rio de Janeiro and São Paulo, Difel.

BASTOS, C. (1991) 'Ciências Sociais e Epidemiologia', *Boletim Pela VIDDA*, 9, 6–7.

CARRIER, J. (1985) 'Mexican Male Bisexuality', *Journal of Homosexuality*, 11, 75–85.

CARVALHO, M.I., *et al.* (1987) 'HIV Antibodies in Beggar Blood Donors in Rio de Janeiro, Brazil', *Instituto Oswaldo Cruz*, 82, 587–588.

CASTRO, B.G., *et al.* (1987) 'Human Immunodeficiency Virus Infection in Brazil', *Journal of the American Medical Association*, 257, 2592–2593.

COHEN, M. (1991) 'Changing to Safer Sex: Personality, Logic and Habit', in P. AGGLETON *et al.* (eds), *AIDS: Responses, Interventions and Care*, London, Falmer Press, 19–42.

CORTES, E., *et al.* (1989a) 'HIV-1, HIV-2, and HTLV-I Infection in High-Risk Groups in Brazil', *The New England Journal of Medicine*, 320, 15.

CORTES, E., *et al.* (1989b) 'Seroprevalence of HIV-1, HIV-2, and HTLV-I in Brazilian Bisexual Males', Fifth International Conference on AIDS, Montreal.

CORTES, E., *et al.* (1989c) 'Seroprevalence of HIV-1, HIV-2, and HTLV-I in Male Prostitutes in Rio de Janeiro, Brazil', Fifth International Conference on AIDS, Montreal.

CORTES, E., *et al.* (1989d) 'Study of HIV-1, HIV-2, and HTLV-I in Female Prostitutes in Brazil', Fifth International Conference on AIDS, Montreal.

COSTA, T. (1986) 'AIDS deixa Grupo de Riso e Atinge Mulher e Criança: Bissexuais são Reponsáveis pela Disseminação indiscriminada do Vírus', *Jornal do Brasil*, 14 December.

COSTA, J.F. (1992) *A Inocência e o Vício: Estudos sobre o Homoerotismo*, Rio de Janeiro, Relume-Dumará.

DA MATTA, R. (1983) 'Para uma Teoria da Sacanagem: Uma Reflexão sobre a Obra de Carlos Zéfiro', in J. MARINHO (ed.), *A Arte Sacana de Carlos Zéfiro*, Rio de Janeiro, Editora Marco Zero, 22–39.

DANIEL, H. (1985) 'A Síndrome do Preconceito', *Comunicações do ISER*, 4, 48–56.

DANIEL, H. (1989) *Vida Antes da Morte*, Rio de Janeiro, Tipografia Jaboti.

DANIEL, H. and MÍCCOLIS, L. (1983) *Jacares e Lobisomens: Dois Ensaios sobre a Homosexualidade*, Rio de Janeiro, Achiame.

DANIEL, H. and PARKER, R. (1991) *AIDS: A Terceira Epidemia*, São Paulo, Iglu.

FATAL, P. (1988) *INVICTA, AIDS Aqui*, Rio de Janeiro, GAPA-RJ.

FINEBERG, H. (1988) 'Education to Prevent AIDS: Prospects and Obstacles', *Science*, 239, 592–596.

FLOWERS, N. (1988) 'AIDS in Rural Brazil', in R. KULSTAD (ed.), *AIDS 1988: AAAS Symposia Papers*, Washington, D.C., American Association for the Advancement of Science, 159–168.

FOLHA DE SÃO PAULO (1986) 'OMS Aletra para Risco de Epidemia de AIDS no Brasil', 6 December.

FOLHA DE SÃO PAULO (1987) 'Entidades Denunciam Violência policial contra Travestis', 10 March.

FOLHA DE SÃO PAULO (1988a) 'Ministro Diz que AIDS Ataca a Elite', 17 July.

FOLHA DE SÃO PAULO (1988b) 'OMS Critica Medida Americana', 29 December.

FONSECA, G. (1982) *História da Prostituição em São Paulo*, São Paulo, Editora Resenha Universitária.

FREITAS, R.S. (1985) *Bordel, Bordeis*, Petrópolis, Editora Vozes.

FRY, P. (1982) *Para Inglês Ver*, Rio de Janeiro, Zahar Editores.

FRY, P. (1985) 'Male Homosexuality and Spirit Possession in Brazil', *Journal of Homosexuality*, 11, 137–153.

FRY, P. and MACRAE, E. (1983) *O Que é Homossexualidade,* São Paulo, Editora Brasiliense.

GAGNON, J. and SIMON, W. (1973) *Sexual Conduct: The Social Sources of Human Sexuality,* Chicago, Ill., Aldine.

GALVÃO, J. (1985) 'AIDS: A "Doença" e os "Doentes"', *Comunicações do ISER*, 4, 42–47.

GASPAR, M.D. (1985) *Garotas de Programa,* Rio de Janeiro, Jorge Zahar Editora.

GEERTZ, C. (1973) *The Interpretation of Cultures,* New York, Basic Books.

GRANGEIRO, A. (1992) 'O Perfil Socio-Econômico da AIDS', presented at the Seminário sobre a Epidemiologia da AIDS no Brasil, Instituto de Medicina Social, Universidade do Estado do Rio de Janeiro, Rio de Janeiro, Brasil.

GRMEK, M.D. (1989) *Historie du SIDA,* Paris, Médécine et Sociétés Payot.

GUIMARÃES, C., *et al.* (1988) 'A Questão dos Preconceitos', *Boletim ABIA*, 3, 2–3.

GUIMARÃES, C., *et al.* (1992) 'Homossexualidade, Bissexualidade, e HIV/AIDS no Brasil: Uma Bibliografia Anotada das Ciências Sociais e Afins', *Physis*, 2, 151–183.

HERDT, G. (1984) 'A Comment on Cultural Attributes and Fluidity of Bisexuality', *Journal of Homosexuality*, 10, 53–61.

Isto é Senhor (1988) 'Vítima do Medo', 14 September.

JOHNSON, E.S. and VIEIRA, J. (1986) 'Causes of AIDS: Etiology', in V. GONG and N. RUDNICK (eds), *AIDS: Facts and Issues,* New Bruswick, N.J., Rutgers University Press, 25–33.

JORNAL DO BRASIL (1986) 'Verbas para AIDS nã\o Acompanham a Incidência', 24 July.

JORNAL DO BRASIL (1987) 'A Doença maldita', 11 January.

JORNAL DO BRASIL (1988) 'Programa da AIDS perde Cz$ 900 milhões', 9 September.

JORNAL DO BRASIL (1989) 'Prostitutas falam de AIDS as Prostitutas', 31 July.

KINSEY, A., *et al.* (1948) *Sexual Behavior in the Human Male,* Philadelphia, Pa., W.B. Saunders.

KINSEY, A., *et al.* (1953) *Sexual Behavior in the Human Female,* Philadelphia, Pa., W.B. Saunders.

KUEBLER-ROSS, E. (1988) *AIDS, O Desafio Final,* São Paulo, Editora Best Seller.

LANCASTER, R. (1986) 'Comment on Arguelles and Rich', *Signs*, 12, 188–192.

LEIBOWITCH, J. (1984) *Um Virus Estranho de Origem Desconhecida*, São Paulo, Record.

MACRAE, E. (1987) 'Os Homossexuais, a AIDS e a Medicina', *Tema Radis*, 5, 41–47.

MACRAE, E. (1990) *A Construção da Igualdade: Identidade Sexual e Política no Brasil da Abertura*, Campinas, Unicamp.

MANN, J. (1987) 'Statement to the UN General Assembly', 20 October, New York.

MESQUITA, F. (1992) 'AIDS e Drogas Injetáveis', *SaúdeLoucura*, 3, 47–53.

MINISTÉRIO DA SAÚDE (1987) *Estrutura e Proposta de Intervenção*, Divisão Nacional de Controle de Doenças Sexualmente Transmissíveis e SIDA-AIDS, Brasília.

MINISTÉRIO DA SAÚDE (1992) *AIDS: Boletim Epidemiólogico*, Ano V, No. 4.

MISSE, M. (1981) *O Estigma do Passivo Sexual*, Rio de Janeiro, Edições Achiamé Ltda.

MORÃES, C. and CARRARA, S. (1985) 'Um Mal de Folhetim', *Comunicações do ISER*, 4, 20–27.

MOTT, L. (1985) 'AIDS: Reflexões sobre a Sodomia', *Comunicações do ISER*, 4, 20–27.

MOTT, L. (1987) 'Os Mêdicos e a AIDS no Brasil', *Ciência e Cultura*, 39, 4–13.

NEWSWEEK (1987) 'An Epidemic Like Africa's: Brazil's Doctors Wonder How Bad AIDS Will Get', 27 July.

NEW YORK TIMES (1985) 'Fright Grips Brazil as AIDS Cases Suddenly Rise', 25 August.

NEW YORK TIMES (1986) 'Brazil Called Lax in AIDS Treatment', 14 December.

NEW YORK TIMES (1987a) 'AIDS in Brazil: Taboo of Silence Ends', 28 October.

NEW YORK TIMES (1987b) 'Brazil, Alarmed, Wars against AIDS', 8 March.

O GLOBO (1988) 'Brasil Carece de Política anti-AIDS', 21 June.

PADILHA, A. (1988) 'Vigilância Sanitária', *Tema Radis*, 10, 5.

PANOS INSTITUTE (1988) *AIDS and the Third World*, Rev. ed., London, Panos Institute.

PANOS INSTITUTE (1990) *The Third Epidemic: Repercussions of the Fear of AIDS*, London, Panos Institute.

PARKER, R.G. (1985) 'Masculinity, Femininity, and Homosexuality: On the Anthropological Interpretation of Sexual Meanings in Brazil', *Journal of Homosexuality*, 11, 155–163.

PARKER, R.G. (1988) 'Sexual Culture and AIDS Education in Urban Brazil', in R. KULSTAD (ed.), *AIDS 1988: AAAS Symposia Papers*, Washington, D.C., American Association for the Advancement of Science, 169–173.

PARKER, R.G. (1989) 'Youth, Identity, and Homosexuality: The Changing Shape of Sexual Life in Brazil', *Journal of Homosexuality*, 17, 269–289.

PARKER, R.G. (1991) *Bodies, Pleasures, and Passions: Sexual Culture in Contemporary Brazil*, Boston, Mass., Beacon Press.

PARKER, R.G. (1992) 'Sexual Diversity, Cultural Analysis, and AIDS Education in Brazil', in G. HERDT and S. LINDENBAUM (eds), *The Time of AIDS: Social Analysis, Theory, and Method*, Newbury Park, Calif., Sage Publications, 225–242.

PARKER, R.G. (1993) 'AIDS, Public Policy, and Political Activism in Brazil', in D. FELDMAN (ed.), *Global AIDS Policy*, in press.

PARKER, R.G. and CARBALLO, M. (1990) 'Qualitative Research on Homosexual and Bisexual Behavior Relevant to HIV/AIDS', *The Journal of Sex Research*, 27, 497–525.

PARKER, R.G. and CARBALLO, M. (1991) 'Human Sexuality and AIDS: The Case of Male Bisexuality', in L. CHEN *et al.* (eds), *AIDS and Women's Reproductive Health*, New York, Plenum Press, 109–117.

PARKER, R.G., *et al.* (1989) 'The Impact of AIDS Health Promotion for Gay and Bisexual Men in Rio de Janeiro, Brazil', presented at the World Health Organization/Global Programme on AIDS Workshop on AIDS Health Promotion Activities Directed towards Gay and Bisexual Men, Geneva.

PATTON, C. (1985) *Sex and Germs: The Politics of AIDS*, Boston, Mass., South End Press.

PATTON, C. (1991) *Inventing AIDS*, New York, Routledge.

PERLONGHER, N. (1987a) *O Negócio do Michê: Prostituição Viril em São Paulo*, São Paulo, Editora Brasiliense.

PERLONGHER, N. (1987b) *O Que é AIDS*, São Paulo, Editora Brasiliense.

PINEL, A. (1989) 'Sexual Behavior Survey of Brazilian Men That Are Clients of Transvestite Prostitutes', Fifth International Conference on AIDS, Montreal.

PIOT, P., *et al.* (1988) 'AIDS: An International Perspective', *Science*, 239, 573–579.

PLUMMER, K. (1975) *Sexual Stigma*, London, Routledge and Kegan Paul.

PLUMMER, K. (1982) 'Symbolic Interactionsim and Sexual Conduct: An Emergent Perspective', in M. BRAKE (ed.), *Human Sexual Relations: Towards a Redefinition of Sexual Politics*, New York, Pantheon Books, 223–241.

POLLAK, M. (1988) *Les Homosexuels et le Sida*, Paris, Editiones A.M. Métailié.

QUINN, T.C., *et al.* (1986) 'AIDS in Africa: An Epidemiologic Paradigm', *Science*, 234, 955–963.

RAMOS, S. (1988) 'A Metamorfose do Sangue na Hora da AIDS', *Tema Radis*, 10, 20–21.

REGAN, M. (1987) 'Brazilian Bishops Split on Strategies to Control Spreading AIDS Epidemic', *Latinamerica Press*, 19, 6.

ROBINSON, T. (1989) 'London's Homosexual Male Prostitutes: Power, Peer Groups, and HIV, *Project SIGMA Working Paper*, 12.

RODRIGUES, L. (1988a) 'Brazil's Educational Programme on AIDS Prevention', World Summit on AIDS, London.

RODRIGUES, L. (1988b) 'Public Health Organization in Brazil', in A.F. FLEMING (ed.), *The Global Impact of AIDS*, New York, Alan R. Liss, 229–232.

RODRIGUES, L. and CHEQUER, P. (1987) 'AIDS no Brasil, 1982–1987', *AIDS: Boletim Epidemiológico*, Ministério de Saúde, Ano 1, No. 6.

SABATIER, R. (1988) *Blaming Others: Prejudice, Race and Worldwide AIDS*, London, Panos Institute.

SAN FRANCISCO CHRONICLE (1988) 'The AIDS Epidemic in Brazil: Blood Transfusions the Main Concern', 7 June.

SANTA INEZ, A.L. (1983) *Hábitos e Attitudes Sexuais dos Brasileiros*, São Paulo, Editora Cultrix.

SIMON, W. and GAGNON, J. (1984) 'Sexual Scripts', *Society*, 22, 53–60.

SONTAG, S. (1977) *Illness as Metaphor*, New York, Farrar, Straus and Giroux.

SONTAG, S. (1989) *AIDS and Its Metaphors*, New York, Farrar, Straus and Giroux.

SULEIMAN, J., *et al.* (1989) 'Seroprevalence of HIV among Transvestites in the City of São Paulo', Fifth International Conference on AIDS, Montreal.

TAYLOR, C. (1985) 'Mexican Male Homosexual Interaction in Public Contexts', *Journal of Homosexuality*, 11, 117–136.

TREICHLER, P. (1992) 'AIDS and HIV Infection in the Third World: A First World Chronicle', in E. FEE and D. FOX (eds), *AIDS: The Making of a Chronic Disease*, Berkeley and Los Angeles, Calif., University of California Press, 377–412.

TREVISAN, J.S. (1986) *Devassos no Paraíso: A Homossexualidade no Brasil, Da Colônia à Atualidade*, São Paulo, Editora Max Limonad.

TURNER, C.F., MILLER, H.G. and MOSES, L.E. (1989) *AIDS, Sexual Behavior, and Intravenous Drug Use*, Washington, D.C., National Academy Press.

VEJA (1985a) 'A Multiplicação do Mal: A AIDS se Espalha', 14 August, 56–69.

VEJA (1985b) 'Primeira Vítima', 4 September, 109–110.

VEJA (1987) 'Hospitais Recusam Pacientes de AIDS', 9 December, 55.

VEJA (1988) 'Morrendo aos Poucos a Cada Dia', 10 August, 66–76.

VEJA (1989) 'A Síndrome revista', 1 February.

VISÃO (1987) 'Único Remédio: Informação', 18 February, 36–43.

WASHINGTON POST (1987) 'Some Victims Wish to Spread AIDS Sparks Fear in Brazil', 4 November.

WATNEY, S. (1987) *Policing Desire: Pornography, AIDS, and the Media*, Minneapolis, Minn., University of Minnesota Press.

WEBB, N.L. (1988) 'Gallup International Survey on Attitudes towards AIDS', in A. FLEMING *et al.* (eds), *The Global Impact of AIDS*, New York, Alan P. Liss, 347–355.

WEEKS, J. (1981) 'Discourse, Desire and Sexual Deviance: Some Problems in a History of Homosexuality', in K. PLUMMER (ed.), *The Making of the Modern Homosexual*, Totowa, N.J., Barnes and Noble, 76–111.

WEEKS, J. (1985) *Sexuality and Its Discontents: Meanings, Myths, and Modern Sexualities*, London, Routledge and Kegan Paul.

WORLD HEALTH ORGANIZATION (1990) 'Update: AIDS Cases Worldwide', *Weekly Epidemiological Record*, July.

YOUNG, A. (1973) 'Gay Gringo in Brazil', in L. RICHMOND and G. NOGUERA (eds), *The Gay Liberation Book*, San Francisco, Calif., Ramparts Press, 60–67.

DE ZALDUONDO, B. (1991) 'Prostitution Viewed Cross-Culturally: Toward Recontextualizing Sex Work in AIDS Intervention Research', *The Journal of Sex Research*, 28, 223–248.

Index

Milton Keynes UK
Ingram Content Group UK Ltd.
UKHW031151141024
449569UK00024B/900